2020
TORN BY
COVID

2020 TORN BY COVID

Dick Armstrong

MILL CITY PRESS

Mill City Press, Inc.
2301 Lucien Way #415
Maitland, FL 32751
407.339.4217
www.millcitypress.net

Paperback ISBN-13: 978-1-66287-452-9
Hard Cover ISBN-13: 978-1-66287-453-6
Ebook ISBN-13: 978-1-66287-454-3

TABLE OF CONTENTS

PRELUDE

2020 PANDEMIC JOURNAL

At the beginning of the COVID–19 Pandemic in January/ February 2020, I personally looked back on worldwide health events, which had impacted millions of lives in every part of the world, not only in my lifetime, but the generations before me, and realized how little I knew about the origin of these diseases or its impact on society. When considering Diphtheria, Sar's, Tuberculosis, HIV, Polio, as well as early childhood diseases, like chicken pox, mumps, whooping cough, measles and etc. I like many other people of the world who were not personally impacted, have little if any recollection of how and where these crisis disease events originated, progressed, how they impacted the world, and how they were ultimately brought under control.

I decided to begin an ongoing recap of the emerging COVID-19 pandemic, and try as best I could to leave a diary of its progression, and its impact on the worldwide community for future generations of not only my family, but others.

When I started this journey, little did I know the impact this disease would have on the world and the people around me. Little did I know the impact this would have on our education system as we knew it, or on our health community, who became stressed beyond its capabilities. Little did I know it's impact on families, who became isolated. Little did I know, grocery shopping would be done on line, and become bags that were dropped off out your front door. Little did I know people desiring medical surgery, would face postponements, as hospitals were delaying surgeries that they determined were elective. Little did I know that our elderly family members, would become isolated in nursing home rooms, with their only family contact through the window in their room, if they happened to have a ground level room, as no visitation was allowed in nursing homes, or hospitals. Seniors facing death in a nursing home, or in hospital care on a respirator, faced the end of life alone. Family members remained distanced from any personal support. For millions of people facing death, their families could only pray, the end would be peaceful, and they left knowing they were loved.

The impact of 2020 is, and was, felt by every american, and every citizen of the world. No one of our generation, would ever live through a period of life, like 2020.

IT WAS A YEAR

TORN BY COVID

The History of Covid-19, The Beginning

In early 2020 the World entered a period of devastation not seen in many of our lifetimes. On 12/31/2019 China advised the World Health Organization, (WHO) that the population in Wuhan China, was experiencing evidence of a new virus similar to the SARs Virus from 2003. It was rapidly moving through the population of Wuhan's 11 million people, and no cure, or preventive measures were known to slow the progression of this virus. A virus, unlike a bacterium, is very fragile and not a living organism, and thus it cannot be killed.

Wuhan is a major manufacturing city for worldwide companies that produce in China. They export products worldwide, and typically have in their city, scores of worldwide business personnel in residence, and business visitors from countries all around the world. As the virus evolved and began to spread in Wuhan, these non-residents quickly felt the need to vacate this area, and return home. No one at that time realized that when they were leaving, potentially they were carrying with them on the plane, the virus, which would ultimately infect the entire world. It was the beginning of COVID-19.

This virus, was determined to be spread through droplets from humans. A sneeze, a cough, mouth spray while talking, could be passed and remain on another person, eventually causing breathing issues requiring hospitalization, and possible death. Early on, it appeared the older population, and people with health issues were the most vulnerable. This continued to be the profile of the virus as it moved across the world. Eliminating contact with anyone who had potentially been exposed to the virus, was the only logical direction to pursue. China began closing factories as infections and deaths skyrocketed. Isolation became the norm and appeared to be the only way to slow the spreading and reduce the daily death count.

This virus was completely unique from other known recent contagious infections. In most cases contact tracing can typically trace the progression of the infection sourced, but in the case of COVID-19 the progression is a speed demon. It's not just that it is contagious, but how it's contagious. Ebola for example isn't contagious until someone is seriously ill. Tuberculosis, which is a respiratory disease, takes weeks, or months to cause symptoms, and It's not spread until they are symptomatic. The flu, which early on people were trying to make comparisons, causes symptoms in about two days, and rarely more than four days. You might be contagious, but the number of contacts is probably limited to a single day. COVID-19 has its own infectious rules. Symptoms usually arrive in two to four days, but can be as long as two weeks. The virus lodges in the sinus and throat, where it's expelled by breathing and talking, and can be infecting others. The virus doesn't reflect the telltale signs such as fever and dry cough, until it's made its way into the lung's days later. Also, the first 24 hours after symptoms typically appear, were lost due to slow ability to test and to confirm contamination. The world was totally unprepared for the potential magnitude of this crisis, even though pandemics were not unknown to the worldwide medical community.

HISTORY OF PANDEMICS

Since the beginning of time, the world has encountered diseases that impacted virtually every populated area of the world. What could be a comparative basis for the progression that was happening in 2020, is the 1918-1919 flu pandemic, aka Spanish Flu. It was the deadliest global epidemic since the black death plague, and was rare among flu viruses for striking down the young, the elderly, and the healthy. In the US, this pandemic lowered the average life expectancy by 12 Years. Infectious disease experts have for years contended the base of this virus from 1918-19 never really went away. After infecting an estimated 500 million people worldwide (a third of the global population at that time) this H1N1 strain hung around and became the basis of the regular seasonal flu, in various forms worldwide.

But every once in a while, direct descendants of the 1918 flu virus, combines with a bird virus, or swine virus, which is what happened in 1957, 1968, and 2009. In 1957, the Hong Kong flu spread throughout China, and then the US, causing 14,000 deaths. A second wave followed in 1958 causing 1.1 million deaths globally. In 1981 the HIV virus is believed to have started with Chimpanzees in west Africa, and then spread throughout the U.S. Since its inception, about 35 million people have died of the HIV aids virus.

In the 1918-1919 Pandemic, Mask-Wearing rules met with great resistance, as well as other government mandates, as they tried to initiate restrictions to control the virus. Schools were closed as were businesses, and churches. Ultimately 50 million people died, of which 675,000 were in the US. There continued at that time to be great resistance to Government imposed restrictions.

As the 2020 virus was starting to spread out of control, countries began to struggle dealing with a new virus which could potentially completely wipe out the human population. Never before has the entire World-wide community faced a pandemic with the magnitude of this out-of-control virus, with no remedy in sight. In early 2020, Cruise ships around the World, became carriers of infected passengers, as they were unaware at that time, of the potential serious issue facing the world. They continued picking up passengers, and disembarking passengers at worldwide ports. As passengers became ill, and sickness spread among the passengers and crew of the cruise ships, and infections began to be identified as COVID-19, attempts to dock at their scheduled ports, was denied. The Port cities were totally unprepared to treat the passengers and crew who had tested positive with COVID-19.

Cruise ships in an attempt to deal with the recommended worldwide treatment, initiated passenger isolation in their cabins, for a 14- day period. Passengers locked themselves in their cabins with meals delivered outside the doors. Ships cruised at sea to meet isolation requirements. When docking was finally permitted, the passengers with residency in the country of disembarkation were departed first, and sent to quarantine in that state. Other passengers exited the cruise ships, and were taken by Government transportation to

Military installations for 14-day Quarantines. Two cruise ship companies sent vacant ships out to sea, to meet others of their fleet, and transfer deceased and seriously infected passengers, in an attempt to separate infected people from the other passengers.

The Panama Canal closed passage to ships, but later reopened due to worldwide pressure, as ships needed to obtain passage to be able to meet the needs of the infected and deceased passengers. The cruise Industry came to a complete halt worldwide.

UNITED STATES

The U.S. progression began mid-February 2020 as Americans visiting Wuhan returned. Initially, major infection areas were Seattle, L.A., and NYC.

It spread quickly and total infections by April 1st 2020 in the U.S, totaled over 250,000 people and 6,900 deaths, with record infections and deaths being recorded daily. NYC alone accounted for over 2,900 deaths. One week later on April 6th infections in the U. S. exceeded 300,000 people and the death toll was over 8,100 people., A total of 3,500 was reported in the State of New York, of which 1,900 were in NYC. Never before had the U.S experienced anything of this magnitude and they were totally unprepared. Massive numbers of protective gear and equipment was in immediate demand, and production of these elements was months away. The U.S. at this stage of the Pandemic, had knowledge of the progression and its impact, and had an opportunity to move ahead of the virus and implement a plan to help protect the Americans.

The U.S. leadership discounted the severity of this disease and failed to respond to the Medical and the Scientific community. The Leadership of the administration failed the American people, while other nations were aggressively addressing the impact of this virus on their people. With no known cure or vaccine available, cites and countries began to mandate individual quarantine, and social distancing. People were urged, then required to remain in their homes. Businesses were to remain closed unless you were deemed part of the essential community. Grocery, Drug, and other select businesses, were to remain open. Malls were closed, restaurants, and bars, were closed. Concerts, and sporting events were cancelled. No NBA, NHL, or MLB opening day. Wimbledon Tennis was cancelled, as were the Summer Olympics in Japan. The world was moving to a standstill. Over 10 million people became unemployed in the U.S the last two weeks of March. People were limited to groups of no more than 10 people, and requested to maintain a 6-foot separation. People were allowed to take walks outside but requested they maintain social distancing. Weddings were cancelled. Funerals were delayed until a point in time where people could gather. Schools and Colleges virtually across the country were closed, and on-line classes in homes became the norm for all ages. For a world who in 2019 had record employment, record stock market gains, and were living the dream, reality set in, and within 3 months, the world had dramatically changed.

The Medical community became strained beyond belief. The demand for available beds, the amount of protective gear for staff, and respirators, were in demand in every city in every country. The economies and Governments became strained beyond belief. The daily death numbers from around the world and in the U.S., were staggering. The death rate among senior citizens, due to COVID as well as other health issues, became the highest % of COVID-19 deaths. Senior housing and senior health care facilities were becoming high death rate facilities. To make things more difficult for family with family members in long term care facilities, visitation was not allowed. Family members could not visit and they remained in isolation with food trays dropped off at their doors, by masked health care workers. Health care workers were at a premium and forced to work under very difficult conditions, with an unknown virus and no apparent cure, or vaccine available. Hospitals began to limit surgeries on a need only basis, reducing elective surgeries virtually Nationwide. The worlds health care community was at the most critical stage in history.

THE WORLD APRIL 1ST
3 MONTHS SINCE THE ONSET

As the travelers from Wuhan China returned back to their home countries, the virus spread at an uncontrollable progression. By April 1st, countries around the globe had closed their borders. Air travel between countries became nonexistent. Over 100 countries were struggling to contain the transmission of this disease,

APRIL 1st

Over 1 million people were diagnosed with the virus.
58,000 deaths, 5,000 to 8,000 reported daily worldwide.

Progression in Europe

ITALY–14,700 deaths.
FRANCE – 1,000 deaths in one day to 6,500.
ITALY, SPAIN, and FRANCE combined have 32,000 deaths.

THE WORLD ONE WEEK LATER

Over 1.1 million people infected.

63,000 Deaths.
ITALY- 15,362 Deaths
FRANCE – 7,560 Deaths
ITALY, FRANCE, AND SPAIN,–34,560 Deaths.

By the 2nd week of April, 1.4 million were confirmed infected, with 79,000 confirmed deaths and the progression was growing at uncontrollable levels. In China, where this COVID19, apparently started, restrictions began to be lifted, as numbers of infected and deaths began to drop. A record daily low of 30 new cases reported and 5 deaths, gave hope it may have peaked. Experts would begin to question the validity of the numbers being reported from China, as all information coming out of China is very closely guarded and monitored Their reports were in direct contrast to reports from the rest of the world. Worldwide levels continued to escalate beyond belief. By the 2nd week of April, the toll of deaths in New York City, had exceeded the deaths in 9/11, with over 3,200 COVID-19 deaths. Statewide New York death rates were exceeding 700 per day.

Things continued to progress daily at alarming rates across the world and the U.S. Easter Sunday 2020 throughout the world was a sad desolate celebration. In Rome at the Vatican, St. Peters square was empty versus over 70,000 celebrating a year earlier. The Pope gave the Easter Mass in the Basilica to an empty Church. Churches across the U.S. had services on video into homes. The world had changed and continued to struggle looking for an answer on how to get the country, and economy back on track. Everything remain closed, and people were required to stay home and practice social distancing. Few homes celebrated easter Family dinners. Lives had changed throughout the World and would continue to experience very dramatic change throughout 2020.

Virus confirmations and death numbers from around the world as Easter Sunday ended, was a Holy week like no other. A total of 1,980,900 people had become infected since January 1st, with over 125,000 deaths. The U. S, which had its first recorded infection January 21st led the world with 603,000 reported cases, and 25,143 deaths. Italy, Spain, and France, also continued to struggle to contain the progress, and reported 44,700 deaths. A one-week escalation of over 10,000 deaths.

Senior confinement facilities around the world reported major outbreaks with Britain reporting over 2,000 nursing facilities with confirmed virus infections.

In the U.S, New York continued as the major outbreak part of the Nation with over 200,000 reported infections and 10,800 deaths. 10 States in the U.S accounted for almost 75 % of the confirmed infections and about 80 % of the deaths

In Minnesota, Easter weekend recorded 194 new confirmed cases of COVID 19 to over 1,600 cases and total deaths to 79 since the early March first confirmed case. The virus continues to attack older people and older residents in long term care facilities. 55 of the 79 deaths in Minnesota were residents of care facilities.

Most of the States continue with residents in Lockdown. Schools, shopping centers, sporting and entertainment events are closed, as are Restaurants and bars. Most of the States have set the end of April as a target date to reopen, but that remains unknown as no cure is in sight. Endless trials and treatments are being evaluated at medical facilities and Universities around the World. But at this point isolation seems to be the best option. The President has plans to consider a reopening as soon as possible, as the economy here, and worldwide is in dire straits. His views are being met with great resistance, as isolation appears to be making progress here, and worldwide. It will not stop the infections, but slow the progress, and that is the major goal of most states and countries around the world,

By the middle of April, the Nation remained on lockdown with pressure from political groups to find a way to re-open as the economy was in a downward spiral. State Governors were trying to maintain control of decisions impacting their state but were being pressured. Coalitions among States were formed as opening moves, needed to be coordinated. The North East and the Western States were working together and most of the country was under the lock down orders until May 4th.

As the outbreak continues to grow worldwide, infection and death rates skyrocket. Worldwide numbers by the middle of April record 2.2 million people infected and over 150,000 deaths. In the U.S, 35,000 deaths and over 650,000 infected were recorded. Its impact on the economy is devastating. Over 22 million people have lost their jobs, with unemployment levels not seen since the depression.

The hardest hit segment in the U.S. and worldwide, are Nursing Homes. In the U.S. over 7,000 deaths are in nursing homes. In New York, 72 Nursing facilities have reported 5 or more deaths in a health center with the virus. The staff at these facilities are overworked, and many lack infection and lacing protective equipment. Many are not showing up for work, and infected staff are in quarantine not able to work. The situation in these facilities continues to snowball downhill. Nursing homes care for about 1.5 million people in the U.S. in about 15,400 facilities and the financial impact of COVID-19 is devastating. Nursing homes have had to spend more money on protective equipment and also technology for interaction among patients, and for families who are unable to make visits. A 72-bed nursing home estimates an additional $2,265 per day on personal protective gear, and an additional $1,500 a day on extra nursing staff.

In an effort to reduce the apparent risks, nursing homes had begun to admit fewer residents. A large portion of their revenue is post-surgical rehabilitation, and with hospitals postponing elective surgeries, this source of revenue was drying up. Nursing homes advocates say the industry will need approximately $15 Billion from the Federal Government to ride out the crisis.

Minnesota which had recorded one of the lowest infections and death rates reported its worst day since the outbreak with 159 new cases reported and 17 new deaths on April 17th and 10 more on the 18th. The spread in Minnesota as an example, which appeared slower than many states, recorded 878 new infected cases and 64 deaths in the past seven days, In North Dakota, where confirmed cases remained low, it took a huge jump when 110 people were reported infected in a Manufacturing facility in Grand Forks. The JBS pork producing plant in Worthington MN, the largest employer in that area, was closed after reporting 77 confirmed cases of the virus. Over 2,000 people are employed at the Worthington facility. Other meat producing facilities faced similar closures. Around the states in the U S. and other countries, production facilities with line crews closely aligned, were susceptible to the virus spreading among the workers and ultimately the public.

In China where the outbreak started at the end of 2019, there has been continual questioning of reporting by the Chinese, and contention's they have purposely underreported the numbers of infected people and deaths. On April 15th after worldwide pressure, the Chinese Government raised their original numbers by over 50%. The outbreak was much worse than was being reported to the worldwide community.

In some Asian countries where the rate of infections seemed to be getting under control, increases again rose, Japan's total infections rose above 10,000 and Singapore had a one-day spike of 942 cases.

By April 21, 2020, the president of WHO stated that the worst may be yet to come. Africa, India, and South American countries with large populations, and people in poor living conditions were vulnerable, as their health system was not equipped for such an epidemic. The Hospitals and the available protective safety equipment were totally unprepared to meet this challenge.

Elsewhere around the world some easement of lock down was beginning to surface. In Germany, Sweden, and Slovakia, cars were about to begin rolling off production lines. In Denmark, selective shops were beginning to open. India eased the world's largest lockdown, to allow some manufacturing and agricultural activity to resume. Italy and France remained under tight lockdown. The World at large remained under threat and isolation.

As April progressed. the U. S case infections increased to over 750,000 cases with over 40,000 deaths. Worldwide the infected cases rose to over 2.3 million cases and over 160.000 deaths. Some countries show stabilization while growth in many others remains out of control.

The key to slowing the growth appears to be massive testing among the population to determine who has been exposed to the virus. Attempts to create testing processes has been slow due to available testing kits and the needed approvals by the federal authorities. The U of M and the Mayo Clinic had been aggressively involved in development of testing procedures, and announced success and now have the capabilities to test up to 20,000 people per day in the U.S.

While managing something of this magnitude, the Pandemic should bring harmony in countries as one would assume working to control this would be a unified effort. But not in the U.S. The political environment appears that not even a devastating worldwide catastrophe can unite our political system. Politics rears its ugly head when a unified direction from States and the Federal management should be in tandem. Opposition party State Governors appear to not receive the same supply levels as those of the party in power involving all protective equipment. Currently there exists major issues between the leadership of the country and the states managing the virus issues. Individual states are facing discord among the people. Major protest groups have developed from people out of work, contending everything should immediately open. The medical community continues to warn that we probably will have a major second wave of the virus in the fall and it may present difficulties beyond our current problems as we will also be dealing with the flu virus and ability of the medical community to deal with both these, could very well be over-whelming. Leaders are under tremendous pressure to deal with the unknown.

Federal guidelines suggest reopening can begin when a state has had 14 days of reduced infections reported. Most States have set May 4th as an opening target assuming they meet the guidelines, but cracks are beginning to develop in any unified plan. Georgia has announced plans to open April 25th without many retail establishments which are currently under lock-down, not meeting the Federal guidelines. Las Vegas Mayor announced she would open the Casino's and recommend the patrons maintain social distancing. Virtually every State is beginning to reevaluate its lock down stipulations.

The Federal guidelines were for 14 days of declining infections before moving to the reopening stage, but Governors were pressured to get their state economies back to work, so Federal authorities could not stop the state decisions. In Minnesota which had been one of the last states with massive infections and aggressive lock downs, announced some return of people to the work force beginning April 27th, but as part of the announcement schools would be closed statewide for the remainder of the school year. On line schooling would continue.

Based on the continual daily and monthly focus on number of deaths, suddenly coming into play was the fact that total deaths have increased significantly during the COVUS-19 death tracking. In fact, worldwide total mortality increased worldwide by an estimated 25,000 over normal death counts since monitoring COVID-19 deaths. Normal death count had major increases in virtually every country, over and above COVD-19 death counts. Contributing factors appear to be cancellation of elective surgeries and reluctance to seek medical care and hospitalization. People were determined to avoid isolation in a hospital at all costs.

As the World moved into the last week of April, a devastating month in most of the world, people were becoming anxious to return to some degree of normalcy. People were becoming agitated by lock down requirements, closures of businesses, and the difficulty of virtual learning by their children with school closures, which in some States will now go through the school year.

Worldwide the COVID-19 death count surpassed 202,000, a conservative number based on non-reporting of nursing home deaths in some countries. In India some relaxation of business closures was welcomed in the small business communities, but malls remained closed. In rural areas agricultural and manufacturing restrictions were lifted to ease the economic plight of millions left jobless by the lockdown.

In sections of Asia, China reported the 10th straight day without a death, although the accuracy of the reporting has been in question since the beginning. South Korea reported only 10 new cases had been reported, which is the 8th day in a row 20 cases or less were being reported. No new deaths were reported for the 2nd day in a row.

In Europe, some relaxation is also being planned for early May. In Spain which has had the strictest confinement regulations, Spaniards will be able to leave their homes for short walks beginning May 2nd. Kids will be getting their first fresh air in 44 days once the ban is lifted allowing them to go outside. They will be allowed to go outside for one hour, adult supervised.

Italy which has the largest number of deaths of the European countries with over 26,600 recorded deaths reported the lowest number since March, with 415 reported deaths.

Italy had been the first western nation to be slammed by the COVID-19 outbreak, and it became increasingly clear something went terribly wrong in the Northern Lombardy region. With their first confirmed case on February 21st, the WHO was still insisting it was containable and not as contagious as the flu. Lombardy has 1/6th of Italy's 60 million people and is the most densely populated region in Italy. It also has more people over 65 and 20% of Italy's Nursing homes, a time bomb for the virus. Not understanding how the virus could present itself, there was a lack of clinical information, on how to treat patients experiencing breathing difficulties. Doctors began treating patients at home as ICU units in the hospitals were immediately filled. After years of medical cuts, Italy had gone into this pandemic with 8.6 ICU beds per 100,000 residents the lowest of the western nations average of 15.6. The at home treatment by physicians became the front line for COVID-19 treatment, with doctors working outside the Hospital system. By the time shutdowns were implemented in the towns making up the Lombardy Region, its impact was devastating. Over 20,000 medical personnel were infected and 150 Doctors had lost their lives. Shutting down and or isolating people met with great resistance, as the Industrial community was not supportive based on the impact of COVID's effect on the economy. This region supports 21% of Italy's GDP. When the National lockdown went into effect on March 7th, it allowed factories to stay open which triggered strikes from workers fearing for their safety.

In attempting to evaluate errors, the home treatment was one identified, as well as the decision to allow recovering COVD-19 patients to recover in nursing homes in an attempt to free up Hospital rooms. Another problem area was a decree March 30th not to transport sick patients over 75 to hospitals for treatment. The number of deaths in Nursing homes remains unclear as there is massive evidence, they are not included in the 13,500 Lombardy region fatalities. These actions together with political and business interests contributed to a progression of something that might have been containable.

Britain had held off any relaxation of lock down with over 20,000 deaths. The death count in Britain does not include nursing home deaths. which is estimated to be in the thousands.

On April 28th Prime minister Johnson returned to work after COVD -19 recovery and spending 3 days in an ICU hospital unit.

In the U.S. heading into the last week of April some States are beginning to revise lock down orders and open different segments of the business community. Georgia and Oklahoma opened salons and barbershops, and spas, and Alaska opened dine in Restaurants with limitations. While some states were reducing restrictions, others were extending the lockdowns from the original dates. Wisconsin which was to end its current lockdown April 17th had it extended to May 26th. People had become outraged and had sent over 6,400 E- mails to the governor in a 24-hr. period. One hair dresser, not allowed to work, e-mailed him saying that he and other news media looked well-groomed on T.V. as evidence someone was breaking State rules.

Neighboring Minnesota has daily death rates increasing. Recent 24hr, period recorded 23 deaths, 22 of which were in long term care facilities. Dramatic increases in numbers of infected people were due in part to expanded testing. The testing worldwide, has become more and more critical. As the lockdowns begin to be lifted, testing procedures need to be in place to support the employees at work. The Minnesota governor announced some reopening of business, for industries which do not have face to face contact. Many restrictions accompany this opening, certainly one of which is the employee agreeing to return, when he is unsure of the risk involved. The Lock down order from the Governor is set to expire May 4th, but many feel it may be extended. Schools are closed for the school year, yearly popular events attracting thousands of people are cancelled. The back to the 50's car show, was recently cancelled. The

Minnesota State Fair is currently in limbo. Similar restrictions are in place worldwide since the new year started.

By the middle of the last week of April, the worldwide infections had surpassed 1 million which had doubled in the past three weeks. 213,000 deaths to date 57,000 of which were in the U.S. which has 4% of the world's population, but currently is recording 25% of the COVD-19 deaths. The good news the past week is that the new cases reported and the number of deaths being reported are beginning to peak and flatten globally.

May 2020

May 1st 2020. 4 months have passed since the first announcement of the outbreak in China. In this 4-month time period, over 220,000 people have lost their lives, with total infections in the millions and growing. Every country in the world has experienced a major change in their lifestyle, their livelihood, and the world around them. No travel permitted to many other countries, varying degrees of lockdown, no sporting events worldwide, cancellation of all events attracting crowds of people, unemployment at record levels in all countries. Deserted streets where the social masses assembled, and uncertainty as to our ability to find a cure, or vaccine to manage the progression.

For families, it was the worst of times. Individuals infected were isolated, any health issues requiring hospitalization, meant total isolation from family as, any visitation by family members was prohibited. In most recorded deaths, these dying people were alone as they passed. No family was allowed to comfort their passing. To make matters more intolerable for family survivors, funerals could not be held for the deceased as gatherings were prohibited. The only comfort for families was to plan for a memorial when life as we knew it returned.

As the world entered this fifth month of the pandemic, countries are struggling to deal with lockdowns, business closures, and a devastating economic outlook. In every country, massive efforts to find cures and means to test virtually every citizen, was the worlds focus. But the world trying to deal with the virus was only part of what the world was facing. The focus on the virus was making the world a much more dangerous place. It would appear, that actions were beginning to surface because countries had so much emphasis on the pandemic, they could catch the U.S. and other countries off balance in dealing with military confrontations. In Asia, China has continued to take control of the south China sea by sinking a Vietnamese ship and sending an oil ship into Malaysian waters. North Korea fired off another round of missiles. Russia resumed buzzing U.S. and NATO aircraft over the Baltic and Mediterranean seas. Only China has an aircraft carrier at sea in the Pacific. The two U.S. carriers in that area are both confined to port with COVID-19 infections. The world which now should be united in purpose, is focused on the impact of the virus as it impacts them, not the world, and not its impact on history.

Every Country has dealt with the virus differently, and implemented different approaches to contain the spreading of the virus. Sweden took a radical approach to control the virus deemed herd immunity through exposure. The strategy was to shelter and sequester all those over 65, and those with preexisting health conditions, heart, lung, and diabetes, while letting the rest of the population naturally circulate and become naturally immune. Once over 60% of the population has gone thru this, you will have herd immunity and the virus will be blocked. One of the advantages of this strategy was you avoid the massive unemployment from the closing of all businesses and avoid the 2nd wave of contamination once the lockdown is lifted.

In Italy, the country hardest hit by the pandemic, restrictions will be eased with millions returning to work. Italy has Europe's largest death toll with over 27,000 recorded deaths. Britain held off on its changes to its lockdown, as the death toll topped 20,000, not including deaths in the nursing homes projected to be in the thousands. In France the lockdown will continue until May 11th.

In the U.S. meat processing facilities began to record extremely high levels of virus contamination, and plants began to close in many states for the safety of the workers. Faced with the implications of this decision and the impact of supplies available in the stores, the President required meat processing plants to reopen with safety measures in place,

States began to reopen business based on individual needs and state progress on numbers of infections and deaths. Massive protests from people demanding we reboot the economy by opening of all business. New York has closed all schools for the remainder of the school year. In Washington State which reported the first case, the Governor has extended the Coronavirus stay home order until May 31st.

In Seoul Korea where employees are programmed to return, the logistics of the return are of grave concern. The population is dependent upon mass transit and the subway system packed with people and social distancing is not possible. The alternative for employees to drive to work, creates a bigger dilemma in traffic congestion, and parking availabilities in the major cities. All major cities must find a way to manage this major transportation change as it begins to reopen.

All of the countries in the world begin to move from lockdown to some resemblance of getting back to a safe managed working environment, but reducing sanctions from a lockdown comes with a price. India experienced the highest single day of infections, as they began to re-open. In Russia new cases exceeded over 10,000 for the first time. The death toll in Britain climbed to that of Italy. Worldwide, the virus has infected more than 3.5 million people and records a death toll of 246,000. The U.S accounts for 60,000 of these deaths, almost 25% of the world's total death count.

Massive efforts are ongoing worldwide to develop medications and vaccines. About 100 research groups are pursuing vaccines with about one dozen in stages of human trial. The world faces a major dilemma when a vaccine is created, and how the distribution will be managed by the global leaders. Will an equitable system be put in place for distribution to the have and have not nations? What will be the timeframe for manufactures to produce an adequate supply, and their role in distribution to meet the needs of the world's population?

Other countries continue to look at Sweden who had taken the herd approach and refused to impose a lockdown to their people. Sweden shares the same goals as every other nation to save lives and protect public health, but is tackling the problem through legally enforced measures and recommendations. Social distancing is being recommended, as is expanded testing, and banning of visits to care homes for the elderly. All Secondary, College, and University courses have been moved to on line, and work at home is encouraged. Sweden is not closing schools for younger children, or day care facilities. There exist no regulations for people to remain in their homes. No businesses have been closed, but restaurants are encouraged to operate within social distancing guidelines. Their strategy is based on voluntary measures and individual responsibility. This makes sense for Sweden, but not for many other countries in the World.

Societies worldwide are much different than Sweden's. The key in Sweden, is a high level of interpersonal trust, and a high level of trust in public officials and authorities. So, the use of recommendations rather than a mandate was not unusual. In the U. S. there is a great deal of mistrust among the societies, and a very poor relationship between the public and elected officials.

Locally, In Minnesota, the original lockdown imposed to run until May 4th, was extended to May 18th with some relaxation of conditions for some small business operations. Restaurants and bars would continue to be closed, but other small non-essential business operations could open with curbside controlled sales. The month of April had a dramatic impact on the progression of the virus in Minnesota. To begin the month of April, 629 cases had been confirmed with 12 deaths from COVID-19. Beginning May 1st. the totals would be, 7,234 infected cases, and 428 deaths. The Governor is under tremendous pressure to bring back more retail activity and open small business. Other states that have opened are seeing increases in virus infections and COVID-19 deaths. The Governor also signed an executive order allowing the health care providers to restart elective surgery procedures and surgeries to begin May 13th, if they have a plan to maintain PPE supplies. Dental offices will also be allowed to see patients. This comes after 7 weeks of closure while they attempted to accumulate the necessary safety equipment needed to maintain a safe surgical facility.

While things are beginning to relax, new issues continue to surface. The massive cases of infections via testing in the packing and slaughter facilities has caused inventory issues at wholesale moving into the retail outlets. Wendy's fast-food restaurants has a shortage of Hamburger, and for the first time cannot meet the needs of customers. Kroger the largest retail chain in the nation is limiting customer purchase of fresh hamburger and pork. Costco has limited purchases of fresh meats to three items.

While many look at the daily death rate decline in New York, Chicago and New Orleans, the reality is the country is in the firm grip of a pandemic, with very little hope of release. As states lifted restrictions, meant to stop the virus, impatient Americans are freely returning to shopping and gathering in groups and returning to bars. As they consume drinks in excess, social distancing becomes nonexistent. Any notion the coronavirus threat was fading away appears to be magical thinking with what the latest numbers and models are continuing to show. Projections and the numbers of infections and deaths will continue to significantly increase daily potentially to 3,000 deaths per day by June 1st.

As the world struggles to develop some vaccine to combat the virus strain originating in Wuhan China, a second strain has been identified originating in Europe and spreading into the U.S and is now the dominant strain since mid-March worldwide. Whenever this new Delta strain appears, it quickly infects far more people than the early strain. Total infections the first week in May now are in excess of 3.5 million people and is responsible for over 250,000 deaths since the beginning of 2020. As the U.S and countries around the world attempt to relax imposed lockdowns, there exists the real potential a second wave is immanent and could exceed the conditions being dealt with today.

Early May, the U. S. continues to be the World leader in total infections and recorded deaths. Some would argue data from many countries is inaccurate and under reported, but the reality is, our infection and death rate, is far greater than other countries. Our lack of decisiveness early on and poor federal Government management, put this country behind the world in being prepared to test, and to provide states with adequate PPE, and a defined plan to manage anything this massive. It turned out to be beyond anyone's wildest dreams, or nightmares.

Families have had to deal with devastating issues never before seen in our lifetimes. The death toll in senior living facilities and nursing represents over 80% of the total deaths, and the lockdown prevents families from planning funerals for an unknown period of time. It also produces a massive problem with the deceased remains, if burial is the family plan. In Minnesota and other states in the U.S., refrigerated warehouses are being leased, as hospitals, nursing homes, and Funeral homes have exceeded human remains storage capabilities.

In addition to the grief of being absent during the final days and hours of a loved one's final moments, was the impact on families during the past few months of isolation and the lack of family centered activities during holidays in holy week, Mother's Day, and upcoming Memorial Day and summer vacation. Life here in this country, and countries around the world have changed dramatically in 2020.

The impact of closure and lockdown is destroying economies worldwide. Pressure continues to build from groups who have resorted to protests to open all business operations. Many countries and States here in the U.S. have resisted massive reopening until some progress is made on a vaccine, or at least testing becomes readily available, which can make business operations and manufacturing plants safe for individuals. While progress is being made on vaccines and drugs to assist patients, a cure is far in our future.

Hospitals here in the U. S. are beginning to get limited shipments of an anti-viral drug, remdesivir which while not officially approved by the FDA is under final study, and can be administered by clinics under an emergency use requisition. The drug has shown to reduce the hospitalization stays by 3 or 4 days. It will continue to be monitored by the FDA and the CDC.

While drug testing continues at a record pace worldwide, so does the efforts to determine exactly how the virus migrates between people. Originally it had a been determined the virus is spread by droplets so the suggested guideline was 6 Ft. as moisture from a person drops to the ground in less than 6 feet. If people maintained a 6 Ft. plus distance it could prevent or reduce contamination. While this became the guideline, studies were created to determine if the virus also existed in an aerosol state and could remain longer and in an expanded area.

U.S. regulators have approved a new type of COVID testing which could be the key to opening the country. The agency announced an emergency authorization for antigen tests. The tests can rapidly detect fragments of virus proteins, and can obtain results in 15 minutes or less. Currently, nasal swabs are tested for the genetic material of the virus, and the testing takes hours and requires specialized equipment for testing. Other antigen tests are being approved on an emergency basis. Currently the testing capabilities are in the 200,000, 250,000 range, far short of what is needed to safely re-open schools, businesses, and churches.

Since the beginning of the Pandemic, PPE supplies have been in short supply or non-existent. Never before has the world been faced with a demand for products in quantities, at the same time. The States, Hospitals, Governments, Military warehouses became depleted virtually all at the same time. Warehouses worldwide who had supplies began to search for the highest bidder. Companies who were able to remain open and produce masks, gloves, and gowns began production at record levels, just to fill immediate pipeline needs. States were using 750,000 to 1 million gloves, and over 100,000 masks, and 50,000 gowns in hospitals. This does not include the needs of nursing homes, and business establishments which could remain open. Reserves disappeared almost overnight. Hospitals were at a crisis. All non-elective surgeries were cancelled. Testing procedures were cancelled. Emergency rooms were vacant as people were in lockdown. Doctors were furloughed unless COVD related. Mayo Clinic announced that it projected it would lose over 900 million dollars in 2020, even after reducing salaries, cutting staff, and eliminating building projects. Unemployed people were in danger of losing health benefits. The healthcare system in this country, and worldwide, faced a threat long term to even provide basic medical services.

States and Countries which had mandated lockdowns and closures, were now faced with how to open, when to open, and what to open. What will be the compliance procedure as manufacturers, businesses, churches, schools, re-open? Here in the U.S. the States were given the directive by the Federal Government to meet certain progression guidelines prior to re-opening. As is the case on everything anyone does, the political system comes into play. The party in power is not going to fairly distribute the support as needed, if someone sees a political advantage. That's the case in Minnesota and Wisconsin.

In Minnesota, some restrictions were lifted, but bars and restaurants were to remain closed. Small businesses were permitted to reopen with set guidelines. Churches, group gatherings were to remain closed until June, but Malls were allowed to open May 18th. The decisions were made by the Governor based on executive powers they could use, and did not have to be agreed to by the opposing party. So, the opposing party promptly defeated a bonding bill in defiance. As in most States, decisions became political issues of managing the pandemic, face masks, vaccinations, all had differing points of view.

In Wisconsin the Governor chose to open everything. Such is the case across the country and in many other countries. Some things open, in one state or country not so in others. The openings come at great risk according to the Models of new infections and pandemic.

The U. S. has the largest outbreak in the world with close to 1.5 million cases and about 85,000 deaths. The U.S. now has conducted about 9 million tests beyond others in the world, but was the last to respond to the need to get started. Some countries that locked down in early March and reopened, are experiencing increases in infections and deaths and renewing safety measures.

Midwest Coalition of States mid May 2020

State	Pop.	Millions	Postive Cases	Deaths	Stay at home expires
MN	5.6	125,000	13,000	638	May 18th
IL	12.7	490,000	84,698	3,792	May 30th
IN	6.7	155,000	25,473	1,482	May 18th
MI	10	309,000	49,000	4,714	May 28th
OH	11.7	225,000	26,000	1,483	May 29th
WS	5.8	128,000	10,900	421	May 15th

As the numbers of tests by State continue to increase, the

number of infections also dramatically increase. Deaths continue to record daily highs in most areas. As has been the case, nursing homes and senior facilities record 80 to 90 % of the recorded deaths. This is universal, older people particularly those with preexisting health conditions remain at risk.

As the reopening date approached in many areas of the world, two sporting events occurred for the first time without spectators. A PGA event was held in Florida with no access for anyone other than participants. Proceeds from the event went to COVD-19 relief and over 5 million was raised for COVID relief. Network T.V. carried the Tournament, and it appeared successful other than lack of fan support. Daytona held the first NASCAR racing event on May 17th also with an empty race track stadium. Race car teams were limited to the number of people admitted for support of their individual drivers. These two events without fans were the face of what was coming worldwide for sporting and entertainment events.

May 18th was a target date for many countries to either open or begin to partially open closures and lockdowns. Many countries, and States in the U.S, had the loosening of restrictions tied to progression of safety equipment, and testing and tracking ability. While progress was being made, many were short of original progress expectations. Italy which had been reducing restrictions and was set to reopen bars and restaurants on May 18th, had not met its goal of massive distribution of low-cost masks, an antibody testing pilot project, and a contact tracking app, delayed reopening with massive protests. Many countries are aggressively pursuing a contact tracking app but are running into numerous privacy issues. France was dealt a setback when a Constitutional Court threw out part of the virus tracking law, and ordered the Government to take extreme caution to protect individual privacy rights. France has committed to expand current testing to up to 700,000 people per week.

Individual rights worldwide, suddenly creates barriers, making it difficult to manage a universal process. Tracking of infected individuals and their recent contacts, became difficult to manage with privacy issues in worldwide democracies.

Britain which has Europe's confirmed death rate at over 33,000 has ramped up its testing to over 100,000 per day. It abandoned its contact tracking after the virus overwhelmed its capacity to follow up on the extent of the process. Spain has not resolved the privacy issues and does not currently have tracking in place. Germany has engaged more than 10,000 people in contact tracking, and contends it is part of their lower death rate. Turkey credits its 5,850 teams that have reached out and tested 470,000 people suspected of being infected.

As States and countries begin to open, the risk attached to opening is very high. Too many age groups lack common sense and put themselves and others at risk. It's imperative as the world begins to reopen, people understand it's a different world, and will be for the remainder of some of our lifetimes. The wearing of Masks as we open countries/cities/states, should be a requirement, not an option. Distancing and group requirements need to be maintained, Life as we knew it has dramatically changed. Waiting for the magical vaccine may never happen. While people pride themselves on being independent, May 18th 2020 may be a good time to re-evaluate the concern for others and the world as a neighborhood.

As the world looks ahead to June 2020, and the U.S. enters the Memorial Day weekend, things are beginning to change in terms of lockdown regulations. Testing, which was virtually impossible to manage and make available to the masses is now readily available. The impact of expanded testing results has produced daily record increases in infections. PPE supplies which have been a problem worldwide since the outset are beginning to catch up at all critical levels. While protective equipment is beginning to meet the needs of critical care workers, unthought of items like body bags, have become a massive problem for Funeral directors, who attempt to maintain the dignity of the deceased, and to protect workers handling the deceased. In many cases, body bags are being used three of four times. Directors are wrapping the remains in a product called plastic casket when body bags are not available. To further complicate the death process, delayed funerals are causing a backup of remains, and lack of storage facilities. Many areas are constructing temporary storage facilities to free up morgue space and add to Funeral home capabilities.

All 50 of the U.S. states have crossed an uneasy threshold by beginning to open in some way, but there are vast variations on how states have decided to open up. The opening up of society as we know it, deals not only with the business community, which has basically been shut down for two months or more, but beaches, state parks and amusement areas. People have been out of work and isolated in their homes for over two months, and are pressuring the respective Governors to open their state. Countries around the world face the same dilemma. With no magic formula of what to open and when to open, there will be areas of the world that open too soon, and areas of the world that are too conservative. The Federal guideline in the U.S. was to have a downward trajectory of infections for a 14-day period before reopening, but many states are reopening while falling far short of meeting those guidelines.

Connecticut raised lowered flags to full staff to signal a return to business. Alaska is planning to revert back to full capacity. In Kentucky plans were to open all small business. In the northeast things were progressing at a slower pace. New York was proceeding with a regional opening excluding New York City. In Washington D.C. a stay-at-home order is in effect until June 1st. In Georgia where businesses have been open for a month requiring social distancing, the number of new cases has remained the same or less. Mississippi saw its largest single day increase the day after the state began to reopen. Wisconsin previously made a state wide opening with few restrictions, while across the river in Minnesota, announcements were made with some limited openings on May 25 and follow up reductions June 1st. Restaurants would be allowed to open outdoor seating with numbers and space requirements. Indoor seating would be further reviewed June 1st. Restaurants would require masks for customers and employees with 50% capacity restrictions and table distancing. Barbers and Hair stylists will be allowed to open June 1st. with masking and number restrictions. To avoid major unmanageable crowd control, an announcement was made the 2020 Minnesota State fair was cancelled. This annual state tradition attracts 2 million visitors each year and has run continuously since 1947 when the only closure was the polio epidemic which forced cancellation.

As part of the re-openings Churches were not included. This brought major protests from the Catholic Archbishop and the head of the Lutheran Evangelical Church who indicated they would reopen regardless of the Governors decision. Discussions were held in which a compromise was reached, which would open churches with restrictions. Churches would be limited to 25% of capacity and a maximum of 250 people. Members older than 65 would be encouraged to continue to worship via virtual service.

Minnesota has aggressively tested since May 1st an average of 5,000 people per day. Since May 1st. Minnesota has added more than 15,000 coronavirus cases and 509 fatalities. On Saturday of Memorial Day weekend 840 new cases were reported bringing the state total to 19,845 infections and 852 deaths from COVD-19. 200 of our long-term care facilities have reported outbreaks and over 80% of the state deaths are from long term care facilities. While the daily news is depressing as businesses face major problems, bike shops and bike repair business is at record levels. People wanting to get out, get exercise, are buying bikes and getting old ones out, that need repair and stimulating record growth.

Worldwide openings continue to proceed with caution and restrictions. As some of the World gains progress, new problem areas surface. In Mexico City massive new infections are surfacing and Brazil has become the new contaminated area of the world, with 347,000 cs. The U. S. President has imposed a travel ban on Brazil. Previously travel bans have been put in place from the United Kingdom, Europe and China.

The U.S leads the world in confirmed cases followed, by Brazil and Russia. France is relaxing its border restrictions and allowing migrant workers to reenter and visit family members from other European countries. In Italy for the first time in months, the faithful gathered in St. Peters square for the papal blessing while keeping their distance.

While the world deals with managing the reopening of countries, a massive effort is underway to develop a vaccine which will be available by 2021. Labs around the world continue to work with cautious optimism. Vaccine development typically takes many years, sometimes decades to develop, so to develop a vaccine in a twelve-month period is unheard of. If it actually happens, it will be the fastest vaccine development program in history. More than 100 teams around the world are taking aim at this virus from multiple angles. The development of this vaccine is only the first hurdle, producing the quantities needed to vaccinate the world's population with possibly two doses could require up to 16 billion doses.

In some recent testing, studies were evaluating DNA for possible links as to why some infected people have mild cases while others become deathly ill. Studies are underway to develop possible statistical links between the COVID-19 and genetic variations. One variation in the human genome is a link between respiratory failure, and a gene which determines blood types. Having type A blood type was linked to a 50% increase in the likelihood an infected patient would need oxygen or go on a ventilator. These studies suggest that unexplored areas may play a role on how we deal with this uncontrolled pandemic.

At the World Health Organization Assembly meeting this week, a proposal was made to adopt a voluntary patent pool, which would put pressure on companies to give up their monopolies on the vaccines they develop. Experts are calling for a "peoples" Vaccine which would be available to all countries free of charge. In a world which cared for the human race and the well-being of the its inhabitants, that would be an easy decision. In a world which has been centered on greed and power, the likelihood of this remains a dream.

China has used the Pandemic as a means to take advantage of its surrounding geographic area. Whether in employing its military assets against Japan in the East China sea, or pursuing Island building, in the South Chain Sea. Neighbors are too involved in the impact of the Pandemic, to devote attention to these confrontations. China has defused negative reaction by providing tens of millions of masks, millions of testing kits and ventilators to distract attention from these confrontations. It would appear that there is higher priority to dealing with the Pandemic for these countries.

In Wuhan central China, where this Pandemic originated 5 months ago, there is an unprecedented, campaign to screen the entire population of 11 million people. In nearly two weeks approximately 6.5 million have been tested. The goal in China is community wide testing rather than random testing. Laboratories which had been processing 46,000 tests per day are processing 1.47 million per day. The Wuhan Government is committed to leave no person behind and are warning in public announcements, people who refuse to be tested would have their government issued health codes downgraded, potentially limiting their right to work and travel. An announcement of a testing deadline, warned if not completed by the deadline, the cost would be paid by the individual. The complete testing is necessary to regain confidence in this worldwide manufacturing city. The Chinese Government continues to be under major criticism for its reporting, or lack of reporting to the WHO. Early on in January, the WHO was praising China for its early response and it's sharing of the genetic map of its progression. Reports now indicate the organization was fearful of pushing too hard and alienating the Chinese Government. As it now unfolds China withheld critical data on the genome, or genetic map after the government had fully decoded it. Strict controls within the Chinese Health system were largely to blame. It was only released after a Chinese Lab published it ahead of author-ities, on a virology website on January 11th. The WHO has been under major criticism for not being more demanding of information from many countries, and in fact the U.S has proposed withholding its funding to the WHO. Trump cut ties with the WHO blasting them for allegedly colluding with the Chinese to hide the extent of this epidemic.

While the focus remains massive testing, under discussion with the NHI is a proposal which would involve about 50 Medical centers here in the U. S. and perhaps an equal number worldwide for testing experimental vaccines. The proposed tests would involve approximately 20,000 participants, and another 10,000 placebo participants. The logistics of setting up this type of testing is to many, an impossible challenge. First you have to develop a vaccine that appears to meet the necessary possible protections, develop endpoints, i.e.: what will determine success or failure. What does the vaccine prevent? Death? Hospitalization? Symptoms? Who determines the area of control? Getting common consent forms developed and then signed. This process usually takes many months and no country has that luxury today. A race to develop comes with huge risk. When Jonas Salk announced the successful trial of his polio vaccine in 1955, the world heralded a vaccine that could eliminate a deadly infectious disease overnight, but everything did not follow a perfect plan. Botched batches of the polio vaccine, released after the successful trials of Jonas Salk, permanently paralyzed over 200 people and killed 10. Early vaccines against measles, mumps, hepatitis, may be more like a flu type vaccine, which reduces the risk or the severity, requiring a new shot each year. This test process started a new direction beginning in June, when evidence to support genetic implications and Type A blood, appeared more susceptible to contacting the virus. While testing was progressing worldwide, actions dealing with the virus worldwide was getting continual attention.

South Korea is and will now be watched very closely as they open up the country, including schools. They have been widely praised for rapid testing and tracing along with stringent social distancing. South Korea once had the largest number of coronavirus cases outside China with the first case reported in early January and implemented immediate contact tracing for those infected. The world will be watching closely to monitor a possible second wave, especially with school reopening.

Sweden took a completely different approach to dealing with the progression of the virus. They maintained open business and schools, stressed social distancing and let the virus supposedly run its course. It's the herd approach to let the virus sort itself out, infecting the weak, but assuming the stronger will develop anti bodies and defuse the progress. By June 1st as Sweden evaluated the nations decision not to shut down the economy, or the country as other nations had, but rely on the citizens sense of civic duty. Authorities have asked citizens to practice social distancing, but to leave schools, bars, and restaurants open. Only gatherings of 50 or more people have been banned.

The net result of the strategy in Sweden, June 1st, a nation of 10.2 million people, has seen 4,542 deaths, the highest per capita death rates in the world. Nearby countries recorded 580 deaths in Denmark, 320 deaths in Finland, and 237 in Norway. Sweden's death rate is lower at 43.2 per 100,000 inhabitants, than Spain at 58.1 and Italy at 55.4, but higher than the U.S. at 32.1. Neighboring countries are maintaining travel restrictions, with review scheduled in mid-June.

The herd immunity is based on an estimated percentage of people who have been exposed to the virus and developed an immunity to the progression of the virus. While countries have attempted to proceed with this strategy, the herd percentage remains an unknown, as the COVID-19 is an unknown human virus. According to disease experts the disease is not going to rest until 60 to 70 % of the population has been infected unless we develop a vaccine. The population will need to be infected and develop immunity in order to stop the virus spread. It could conceivably get to a point, where we cannot get away from it unless a vaccine is developed, tested, and produced.

June 2020

By June 1st after 5 months of COVID-19, the numbers in the U.S. and worldwide are staggering. Worldwide, more than 6.6 million people have been infected with over 387,000 deaths. The U. S. has the highest % of infections and deaths with 1.7 million people infected and 104,000 deaths. New York is recording 374,000 people infected and 29,000 deaths, The America's have the largest infection rate with 3,085 per million followed by Europe with 2,230 million. Russia reports 450,000 infections with 5,500 deaths. The elderly in virtually every country records the highest % of infections and deaths, with over 80% of recorded deaths from long term care facilities

June 1st brought many re-openings worldwide, as phase II. In some States and countries restaurants will begin to reopen with restrictions, on distancing and servicing numbers. Churches would also begin to reopen with occupancy of 25% of capacity, maximum 250 people. In Minnesota, restaurants could open with outdoor dining, and 50 % capacity with reservations and masks. Servers would also be required to wear masks. This took effect June 2nd. On June 4th the Governor announced Phase III which would be in effect June 10th which expanded the earlier reopening, to allow Restaurants to open indoors with distancing and 50% capacity. Social distancing would be in effect, with reservations and 50% occupancy. Indoor gatherings would be permitted with groups of 10 people and outdoor gatherings of 50 or less. Masks would be highly encouraged. Gyms, personal fitness centers could reopen with 25% capacity. Personal services such as Salons, could reopen with 50% capacity and reservations. Church capacity for worship could increase to 50%. The infection rate and the death count has somewhat stabilized but far from being under control. The infected number in Minnesota, had risen to over 26,000 with a death total of over 1,100.

While the world was united in attempting to control the spread of the virus with social distancing, lock down, and wearing facial masks to con-trol spreading, the Floyd incident in Minneapolis, triggered protests around the world which ignored restriction recommendations. This will undoubtably reflect in new infected cases.

The continuing protests and massive crowds chanting, singing, unmasked, day after day, packed together are upending efforts by Health officials to track and contain the spread of coronavirus, just as those efforts were finally getting underway. A key component of the tracking program was for newly infected individuals to remember and recount everyone they had interacted with over the past several Days in order to alert others who may have been exposed, and prevent them from spreading the disease further. An impossible task if they have been part of a massive gatherings on one of several days. Its further complicated by the Governments plan to slowly reopen businesses, churches, and other organizations after months of stay-at-home orders and other virus preventive measures, and monitor closely with controlled testing. The protests however were outside where the virus will not spread as easily as indoors, and many were wearing facemasks,

In L.A. the mayor announced the COID-19 testing centers were being closed because of safety concerns related to the violent protests. Testing in Minneapolis will be impacted due to damage to clinics involved in the protests along with other destroyed buildings. Other cities have experienced a major setback in the testing process. Reduced testing could give the virus another head start.

And contact tracing is a bigger concern, particularly in the U.S. as many citizens mistrust anything the government is involved in. It's being handled by a government agency who will be asking where they have been, who they have been talking, to and expecting to get full, truthful answers from the individuals. This is a major concern in the black communities, trying to deal with episodes of police violence and longstanding frustrations with how they have been marginalized and mistreated by people who work for government agencies. And these are the communities that have been hardest hit by the coronavirus in the U.S. and most in need of public measures to control it.

By June 10th many states and Countries had made major decisions regarding reopening business, and Industry, and relaxation of travel restrictions. The States in the U.S varied with re openings. New York City for example reopened Retail stores but maintained curb and online purchase pick up only. No customers were allowed to enter and shop the stores. The city had now 100 days of shut down and had experienced over 22,000 deaths. Other States varied on relaxation of restrictions with theme parks and other social gathering events relaxed on numbers, which are recommended for safety. Restaurants reopened in most states with social distancing regulations and masked service employees. Customers in most all cases are encouraged to wear masks as a safety precaution. As the states and countries reopened, the number of infected cases also increased. In any case there is no evidence this is the beginning of the 2nd wave. The reopening is a step towards establishing a new normal. The jobless rate dropped in May as a result of business openings and call back of millions of employees.

In hindsight the U.S, can reflect on numerous failed actions and decisions which cost many lives. As Americans returned from China in early February potential carriers of this deadly disease, they were diverted to a handful of selected cities for screening by the CDC. The arrivals prompted a frantic scramble as the CDC with decade old notification systems, riddled with duplicative records of phone and address information attempted to track the passenger lists, and make local official notifications. When the system went off line in mid-February, local officials listened in disbelief to the response of the CDC, that some infected passengers are probably getting away. "Just let them go" was the response. Long considered the world's premier health agency, major testing mistakes were made which persist today as the country prepares to reopen. It failed to report active accurate data due to its aging technology and fractured reporting systems. And most important it hesitated in absorbing the lessons of the other nations who were ahead of the U.S. in the outbreak. They let us down was the outcry from most state health officials. There was complete lack of response, and management from the CDC. The network of local and State health departments, hospitals, government agencies, and suppliers were totally unprepared for the speed, scope, and ferocity of the pandemic.

Overseas, the pandemic had moved at different speeds with varying control efforts and results. Japan has kept its death count low despite an early series of missteps. They bungled a cruise ship quarantine and were slow to close its borders, but they record a low of 900 deaths, which is 7 per million people. This compares to the U.S. with 320 deaths per million people and 550 deaths per million in Italy and Britain. Many theories as to why the lower infections. The Japanese have long been wearing masks as a preventive measure. They bow rather than shake hands and Japan began an early campaign of the three C's to get the public to avoid high risk environments. Close contact, closed settings, and crowded places. became instilled in the Japanese culture. While it would appear, Japan was effectively managing the outbreak, hospitals became overwhelmed, and emergency medicine briefly collapsed. Emergency rooms were rejecting patients for admission due to shortages of protective gear, ventilators, and intensive care beds. The handling of the Diamond Princess cruise ship, quarantined in the Yokohama harbor, with 712 of its 3,711 people aboard infected, eventually flooded and overwhelmed the health community. The government has revised its testing guidelines, and is setting up extensive testing stations for early detection of a second outbreak.

As Italy begins to reopen its businesses, the lack of tourism is an issue greater than most other countries. 13.2% of Italy's GDP is tourism. More than 63 million visitors travel to Italy each year and support the 45,000 people who rely on tourism as guides and organizers.

Europe is taking a big step toward normality as many of the countries begin to open their borders to fellow Europeans, after 3 months of lockdown. The border openings are for select countries, including the U.S., and Asia. Latin America, and the Middle East are not included in the Europe border reopening. The openings are to assist the nations to reap some benefits of the upcoming tourist season which begins soon. Greece is one country watching very closely the impact of new travel as they have one of the lowest death rates of any country, 183 overall. Spain which is one of the hardest hit countries is opening June 21st by allowing thousands of Germans to fly to its Balearic Region for a trial run waving a 14-day quarantine for the group. Germany and Poland opened their adjoining borders as did France, but France is requiring British residents to quarantine for two weeks. Demark is opening, but only for tourists from Germany, Norway, and Iceland. Norway is keeping its border with Sweden closed, as are most other countries who are not opening to travel from Sweden as it is viewed as very risky. As Europe opens its borders to neighboring countries, international travel remains banned. In the South America region, reopening continued in Brazil and Mexico, despite cases climbing in the two largest Latin American countries, where officials struggled with its impact on an already weak medical system.

Constant vigilance came into sharp focus as China, which had been reporting reduced infections rushed to contain an outbreak in the capital city Beijing. The outbreak was traced to an open-air fish market where 79 cases were reported in 4 days. Inspectors found 40 samples of the virus in the closed market. Elsewhere, South Korea was attempting to prevent a resurgence when 37 new cases were reported linked to entertainment, church gatherings and leisure activities, Russia which reported it was emerging from the virus outbreak reported 8,250 new cases totaling 538,000 infected and over 7,000 deaths.

As States in the U. S. expand reopening, it comes at a cost which many fear could be the beginning of wave 2. The weekend of June 13 /14 recorded record infection levels in 5 States which had aggressively reopened. New cases are trending up in 20 States. Minnesota which has slowly reopened on a structured plan has seen reduced infections and deaths for five continuous days.

The U.S. now has over 2.1 million reported infected cases and over 115,000 deaths.

That was the infection rate and death total June 15th. By June 25th, 10 days later, complacency continues to set in as people are eager to expand their freedom, and the pressure to reopen has resulted in wiping out two months of reaching some levels of stabilization. Infection levels have skyrocketed in many parts of the country beyond record highs from mid-April. On June 25th, the U.S. recorded 34,700 infected cases in one day, to over 2.1 million, and death totals to over 120,000, the highest in the world. While some of the early outbreak hotspots like New York and New Jersey have stabilized, several other states are setting daily record levels. and Hospitals are at maximum capacity levels. Arizona, California, Oklahoma, Mississippi, and several other States are in crisis. Texas which began lifting its shutdown levels May 1st is now in crisis mode in many key cities, with Hospital crisis units at capacity and it has paused any further reopening of restrictions. States which were aggressively reopening are now struggling to determine a redirection to gain control of the spreading virus. Prospects for some miracle slowdowns are a dream claims one expert. We are facing a forest fire with little chance of control. States which reopened on a slower structured pace are realizing a more controlled progression. Death rates in Minnesota have trended into the single digits and hospitalizations are at a manageable level. The Governor cautions more aggressive openings leads to relaxed social distancing, and ignoring of wearing masks. People are eager to resume normal living and ignoring the risks. The younger generation worldwide, see this as an older people risk disease. Even though the death % is in the 80 to 89 age range, all ages are at risk.

Recent sporting infection cases, would indicate all ages and people are potential to get the virus. Recent Tennis news reported, Novak Djokovic and his wife tested positive after participating in an exhibition match in a tour event in Croatia, and Serbia. Grigor Dimitrov, Borna Coric and Victor Troicki also tested positive. This would appear to potentially delay the opening The Tennis Tour here in the U.S.

Clemson University in the U.S. reported 23 of their Football players who were reporting for Physicals, tested positive, as did three staff people in campus testing. No one has been hospitalized but are in a quarantine status.

As the poor countries around the world continue to beat back the coronavirus, they are unintentionally contributing to fresh explosions of illness and death from other illness. This spring when children were to gather for inoculations, they were suspended for pandemic controls. Not only were vaccines halted, but flights with inoculation supplies were diverted. At risk is the future of a hard fought 20-year collaboration that has prevented 35 million deaths in 98 countries around the world and reduced mortality in children by 44%. Of the 29 countries that suspended measles shots 18 are reporting outbreaks. 178 million people are at risk of missing measles shots in 2020. There were nearly 10 million cases of measles and 142,300 deaths. The same risk exists with other vaccines worldwide for polio, Cholera, tuberculosis, and Ebola.

By June 22nd, more than 8.7 million cases had been reported worldwide with over 462,000 deaths. On June 22nd, The WHO reported over 183,000 cases worldwide the highest single day total, with Brazil, the U. S. and India the top three recorded case numbers. Brazil had 54,700cs, followed by the U.S, and India with 36,700. And 15,400 respectively. In Iran recent testing results record the largest single day spike in cases. Iran reported its first case and death in mid-February and implemented closures in the entire country. Recent relaxations to the closures to celebrate the recent Muslim Holiday had the population become complacent on masks and social distancing. Numbers had risen to 3,500 cases per day but trending down to Around 2,000. This appears to have changed direction. Testing has significantly increased to over 25,000 tests per day, some 1.3 million of the 8 million inhabitants.

The human body is a citadel that relies on the immune system to defend it. A virus is an attacking army that does everything it can do to overrun those defenses. Vaccines cannot prevent the virus from causing an infection, but they can control the infection before it leads to symptoms and disease. Vaccines teach the body to create a specialized force of white blood cells and antibodies that are called up in the event of a life-threatening attack.

Nearly 160 COVID-19 Vaccines are in the development stage around the world today. Although all approaches are distinct, they are based on a few simple strategies, some of which have been around for years. Some are using the entire SARS-CoV-2 coronavirus to induce a broad immune response. But these are difficult to create and production is time consuming. They are often grown in chicken eggs, so millions of hens would be needed to produce worldwide distribution and working with a live virus is risky. Another approach is to take active virus, kill them so they can't replicate and inject them, which prompts the creation of anti-bodies. Many others are focused on development of a synthetically produced S protein and injecting it into the body to induce an immune system to attack the coronavirus. The entire research is in uncharted waters and no quick fix is in the foreseeable future

THE VACCINE TESTING PROCESS

THE DEVELOPMENT FROM LAB TO CLINIC

PRE-CLINICAL TESTING- Scientists give the vaccine to animals to see if it produces an immune response.

PHASE 1 – SAFETY TRIALS- Scientists give the vaccine to small number of people to test safety and dosage, and confirm it stimulates the immune system.

PHASE 2. – EXPANDED TRIALS- Scientists give the vaccine to hundreds of people split into small groups, such as elderly and children to measure differences in reaction.

PHASE 3. – EFFICACY TRIALS – Scientists give the vaccine to thousands of people to see how many are infected versus a placebo group.

APPROVAL – Regulators in each country review the trial results to decide whether or not to approve the vaccine.

OPERATION WARP SPEED – The U.S Government selects five vaccine projects to receive billions of dollars to support development before the vaccines actually are proven to work.

COMBINED PHASES- Some vaccines could be in more than one of the phases.

VIRUS DEVELOPMENT WORLDWIDE

<u>WHOLE – VIRUS VACCINES</u>. Using a weakened or inactivated version of the virus to provoke an immune response

SINOVAC- A State owned Chinese Company currently preparing for Phase 3. trials in China and Brazil. They are currently building a facility to produce 100 million doses annually.

SINOPHARM – A State owned Chinese Company which has started Phase 1, and Phase 2, trials on two inactivated viruses. They are building a facility in Beijing to produce 200 million vaccines per year.

INSTITUTE OF MEDICAL BIOLOGY AT THE ACADEMY OF MEDICAL SCIENCES – Running a Phase 1 trial of an inactivated virus.

<u>GENETIC VACCINES</u>- One that uses one or more of the virus's own genes to provoke an immune response

MODERNA – Part of Operation Warp Speed Eyeing Phase 3. Trials in July.

BIONTECH/PFIZER/ FOSUNPHARMA – A collaboration of a German, U.S., and Chinese company which is part of WARP SPEED who hope to have human trials by fall.

IMPERIAL COLLEGE LONDON/MORNINGSIDE – A plan to start Phase 1/2, Trials to boost production of a viral protein to stimulate the immune system.

INOVIO- Developing a DNA based vaccine that produces antibodies. Safety trials in humans ae underway in the U.S. and will start in South Korea at the end of June.

CUREVAC- A German research company who had success with a rabies vaccine based on an RNA design which passed Phase 1 trials.

VIRAL VECTOR VACCINES – Vaccines that use a virus to deliver coronavirus genes into cells to provoke an immune response.

ASTRA/ZENECA-UNIVERSITY OF OXFORD – Based on a chimpanzee adenovirus. The vaccine is beginning Phase 2/3 testing in England and Brazil. Supported by Warp Speed funding.

CanSinoBIO–A Chinese Company testing a vaccine based on an adenovirus called Ad5. Phase 1 trial date has been published.

BETH ISRAEL DEACONESS/ JOHNSON AND JOHNSON- Testing an adenovirus called Ad26, recently acquired Warp Speed and starting Phase 1/2 in late July.

MASSACHUSETTS EYE AND EAR / NOVARTIS – A Swiss company looking to manufacture a vaccine based on a gene therapy treatment that delivers gene fragments into cells. Phase 1 trials are to begin late 2020.

MERCK – Announced it would develop a vaccine from vesicular stomatitis viruses an approach they successfully used to develop a vaccine for Ebola. Partnered with IAVI and part of Warp Speed.

NOVAVAX – Started a Phase 1 / 2 trial on a vaccine made up of microscopic particles carrying fragments of coronavirus proteins.

CLOVER BIOPHARMACEUTICALS – Developing a vaccine containing a protein taken from coronaviruses.

TEXAS CHILDRENS HOSPITAL / BAYLOR COLLEGE OF MEDICINE – Reviving a concept used by the Baylor development for the SARS EPIDEMIC IN 2002.

UNIVERSITY OF QUEENSLAND – Australia's plan to deliver viral protein to develop a stronger immune response. Phase 1 trials not scheduled to begin until 2021.

SANOFI- A French research company will produce viral proteins using engineered viruses that grow inside insect cells. GSK will supplement these proteins to stimulate the immune system.

VAXART – An oral tablet containing different virus proteins. Now preparing for Phase 1, trials to begin late summer 2020.

July 2020

B y July 1ˢᵗ, Countries around the World were moving up testing procedures, and preparing to aggressively speed up trials. The Virus was finding new victims worldwide in bars and restaurants, offices and casinos, confirming what many scientists had said for months that the virus lingers in the air infecting those nearby. If airborne transmission is a significant factor in the pandemic, especially in crowded spaces with poor ventilation, the consequences for containment will be significant. Ultimately masks may be needed indoors.

By July 1ˢᵗ, most Countries and States here in the U. S. had plans to partially or completely reopen most business operations with some or no restrictions. The State actions here were varied with many aggressively opening in late May or early June while others were cautious and had not completely opened and were looking at July to begin to normalize. While distancing and masks were important factors in the success of the reopening, the younger generation looked at this as an older generation problem, and ignored all forms of control, and as bars opened protective measures were ignored. On June 26ᵗʰ Texas, Florida and Arizona began to retreat, as bars and young infections aggressively climbed within the U.S recording over 40,000 cases in a single day an all-time high. These States joined the small, but growing list of States of those that are either beginning to backtrack or putting any further reopening's on hold because of a comeback by the virus.

With Texas reporting more than 17,000 new cases the last three days of June and a record high of 6,000 in a single day, the Texas Governor ordered all bars closed, and restaurants to scale back capacity. In Florida where over 10,000 cases were reported in a single day, no alcohol is allowed served in any establishment. The patrons were disregarding social distancing and masks were not being worn by the majority of the younger generation. Beaches in South Florida will now be closed for the 4th of July weekend. Test results as positive have risen to 15% from 4 % at the end of May. States like Arizona and Arkansas where the Governors were not requiring the population to wear masks, were recording record infection rates, particularly among the younger generation. Louisiana recorded its second day with over 1,300 new cases and the Governor suspended further easing of regulations. In Nevada, the Casinos and in other public places people will now be required to wear face masks. In California, the Governor rolled back reopening in 19 L.A. counties and ordered bars and restaurants closed immediately. He urged 8 other counties to issue local health orders to mandate the same. Florida beaches will continue to be closed to avoid further spread as interactions among young people are driving the surge in new infected cases. New York which was the virus epicenter has moved to the opposite end of the spectrum with a daily death toll of 5 people versus nearly 800 in April. They still lead the death toll with over 25,000 of the U.S death toll. In the State of Washington, the Governor has put on hold plans to move counties to the 4th phase of his reopening plans.

Worldwide the virus numbers that were be-ing reported was over 125,000 deaths, and 2.4 million infected people, health officials had contended the real number was approximately 10 times larger and death totals were over ½ million people. On June 30th the actual confirmed numbers now being reported were infections of 10 million and deaths exceeding 500,000. About ¼ of those deaths have been in the U.S. by far exceeding any other country in the world. Brazil, is a distant 2nd in the total death count with about 57,000.

When countries were proceeding with reopening plans, based on stabilization of infections, the WHO reported 189,000 cases was reported on June 28th, the highest single day total, eclipsing the 183,000 recorded less than a week earlier.

Here in Minnesota, where openings have moved slowly, the movement to reopen bars has dramatically increased the number of infections, and the % of cases for residents in their 20's. The consensus is if we are going to continue to reopen the economy, the younger generation needs to take this seriously. A dramatic change is taking place in the infection rate, and the impact of complacency to protection of those around us.

The European Union is opening its borders on July 1st to other European countries but will continue to block travel to and from the U.S. and Russia, due what they describe as lack of control of the virus. China will also be included in the reopening, but only if they reciprocate travel to their country. The U. S. banned most EU travelers in early March when the virus was raging in Europe and has not eased its own restrictions since then, even though infection rates have significantly dropped as have deaths. Several countries in Europe continue to push for the opening to American tourists, as their economy is dependent on the tourists from America. Seven Million people from America visited Europe last June – August, and Countries like Italy, Spain and Greece depend on this for their economy. European countries are imposing lockdowns in areas where a spike in infections appear extremely aggressive. In England, the city of Leicester reports a spike in its Asian community, and is facing a lockdown. In Germany lockdowns were renewed in a Western region of 500,000 people, after about 1,300 workers in a slaughterhouse facility tested positive. In Africa rates continue to climb with 375,000 infections confirmed and over 9,500 deaths.

The U. S. is paying the price for total mismanagement of this crisis. President Trump from the beginning did not take this seriously and Americans are paying a terrible price. It has become a huge political issue and the blame game has not helped the cause. Our economy and health system will take years to recover.

As countries attempt to reopen, transportation and its impact come into play. Mass transit is a risk for the bulk of people returning to work and the highway system is not prepared for new increased auto traffic. Biking lanes are continued to be expanded, as cities have imposed fees for autos entering congested inner-city areas. Cities like London, San Francisco, and major cities in South America are frantically working to manage the changes the Pandemic has created.

By the beginning of July, the U.S. and the world had made major efforts to reopen virtually all phases of business and recreation services, Disneyland had reopened, bars and restaurants had reopened with restrictions, and beaches and social gathering had resumed gatherings with relaxed restrictions, namely face masks. But the changes worldwide and in the U, S, in the weeks leading up to July, came at an enormous cost. By July

7th. confirmed cases were on the rise in 41 of the 50 states and the testing cases coming back as positive was on the rise in 39 of the 50 states. Florida which had an early relaxation of control, had an all-time high of 11,400 positive cases in one day, with 18% testing positive also an all-time high. This is six times higher than the count 1 month ago. The U.S. recorded over 50,700 daily new confirmed cases doubling the daily total over the past month and higher than the what the country witnessed in April/May when the crisis appeared to be at a peak. All but 10 states are showing an upswing in new cases being reported. The outbreaks in July with the highest reporting. were the states of Florida, California, Texas, and Arizona, which reclosed or clamped back on bars restaurants, movie theatres over the past weeks. Other states are reporting troubling trends as well. Positive tests have doubled in Georgia, Kansas, Montana, Michigan, Missouri, Tennessee, South Carolina, and Ohio. In Nevada the number of infections has tripled while in Idaho it is 5 times higher.

Texas who in early May began one of the most aggressive reopening's of any state has ordered the wearing of masks in all counties with at least 20 confirmed cases, The number of hospitalization's has tripled since late May. They reported over 10,000 cs for the 4th day in a row and record deaths. In California, the Governor announced new statewide restrictions which will halt all indoor dining and close bars. At the same time Los Angeles and 30 other counties will be forced to close gyms, churches, hair salons and malls. School districts are evaluating their positions and will make fall opening decisions sometime early August. The school openings are a divisive issue with many insisting they reopen, others contending they are putting children at risk.

Mid July major chains such as Target, Walmart, and numerous others are requiring masks be worn by anyone entering their stores. The wearing of masks has become a hot political issue with cities and businesses requiring the wearing of masks, when in fact it's virtually impossible to enforce. In Georgia, the mayor of Atlanta as well as 14 other cities have issued mandates for people to wear masks in public. The Governor has filed a lawsuit against the cities initiating the mandate that he and he alone can make these health decisions for the state. The Atlanta Mayor refuses to change her position, and is enforcing the mandate. Instead of working to develop a plan to protect residents, a political struggle surfaces and residents have become lost in the outcome.

As states face new record infections and deaths, hospitals are stretched to the limit in Texas, Arizona, and Florida, as well as other States with record infection trends. The record death growth daily, has cities out of morgue space for the bodies, and cities are renting refrigerated trailers to accommodate hospitals and funeral homes, who have limited capacity to store the re-mains and are out of space.

Worldwide mid-July, the number of confirmed cases has risen to over 13.5 million people and over 580,000 deaths. 5 days later the totals are over 14 million cases and 600,000 deaths.

Brazil reported the country had passed 2 million confirmed cases and 76,000 deaths. The death rate has risen to over 1,000 per day.

In Europe where vacation plans are in full swing after months of lockdown, scenes of drunken tourists ignoring social distancing, and flouting quarantine measures raised fears of a resurgence of infections. In France which saw an increase in outbreaks, made masks mandatory in public places. India had infection increases to over 32,000 in a day to over a million infections. The popular western beach state of Goa, has reimposed a three-day lockdown and a curfew after recently reopening.

Back in the U.S. Minnesota where the reopening's moved at a very cautious pace, the numbers have not risen to unmanageable levels and daily death rates have been in single digits. Expected further openings targeted for the end of July are on hold pending the lack of compliance in many bars and restaurants. The Governor has issued a warning the current reopening's could change if complaint violations continue to increase. Young people do not appear to take the pandemic threat seriously and rates of infections in the younger age group continue to rise. Currently the age group with the most infections is 20–29 while the age group with the most deaths continue to be the 80–89-year-old. The Governor joined 30 other states with a mask mandate to begin July 25th. Masks must be worn in all public places. This took the pressure off many retailers who were struggling with implementation on their own.

As the end of July rapidly approached, the pandemic continued to escalate, at rates in the U. S and globally that flooded emergency rooms, forcing some patient into hallways due to beyond capacity hospitalization. In Texas which continues to escalate numbers of new cases, Houston had described the current situation as worse than Hurricane Harvey. Texas on the 20th of the month reported over 10,000 new cases for the 4th day in a row. Other states are recording alarming daily infections. Florida recorded 10,200 new cases, and 90 additional deaths. Missouri reported a new high of 968 cases in one day, while Arizona recorded 147 daily deaths. Worldwide the WHO reported a single day infection record of 259,000 new cases. The

U.S., Brazil and India lead with total numbers of infections. In Africa, with 350,000 cases, roughly 1/2 of the cases are from South Africa. The health minister indicates that fatigue seems to have set in, and people have let their guard down with lack of social distancing and face mask abandonment.

Global totals by July 20th total 603,000 deaths with over 14.3 million infected cases reported. These numbers continue to be on the low side as not all countries are reporting the same data and have reporting capabilities. The infections continue to be a major growing issue as complacency has replaced common sense among the world's population. Nations however are beginning to impose a much stricter emphasis on compliance. In Australia, for example a $140.00 fine is imposed for someone not wearing a mask in a public place. The premier states it's about changing habits, making it part of your routine.

As August approaches, many companies involved in the development of a vaccine have shown some positive preliminary results. Scientists at the University of Oxford have partnered with AstraZeneca, to create and produce a protective immune system. Trials have shown a positive response and larger trials are in the process. Once the vaccine has been proven to be effective, AstraZeneca will partner with them to produce and has committed to produce 2 billion doses. The trials will be expanded to other countries as they evaluate the effectiveness, Brazil and South Africa are now in the testing phase.

As the case rate in Minnesota approaches 50,000, the death rate has not skyrocketed as most other states, daily deaths continue to be single digit. The death rate in nursing facilities continues to drop off with the current death rate per week of 13. compared to 137 per week in May. Currently about 77% of the deaths in Minnesota were residents of nursing homes, assisted living and rehabilitation centers. While the rate among these facilities declines, Communities of color disproportionately are affected by the virus. Blacks' hospitalization rates are 346 per 100,000, Hispanic's are 311 per 100,000, while whites have a hospitalization rate of 27.

As July 2020 comes to a close, very little if any optimism is reflected in the U.S. and or Countries Worldwide. In the U.S. over 5 million people have reportedly been infected with over 162.000 deaths. The U.S. continues to be by far the leader in total infections and deaths. The World views the U.S. handling of the pandemic with amazement, as it was mishandled from the beginning. How could the most powerful nation in the world with the benefit of over 4 weeks of time to prepare, as it progressed worldwide, fail to recognize the potential of this pandemic. Instead, our President passed it off as something that would quickly pass. Medical experts were completely ignored and the people blindly accepted this fate, which led to massive infections and deaths and apparent total denial from the key leadership. Europe is hesitant to open borders to Americans with fears they can rekindle a new surge of infections, when many European countries are beginning to see some progress. They see that Italy which was once the ground zero of Europe's epidemic immediately imposed a 10-week lockdown, and now as they're open are a model of viral containment. Their view of the U.S. handling, is as if health of-ficials were not allowed to be heard, the U.S. could have come to grips with this in March and prevented thousands of needless infections and deaths. The Administration continues to defend its position, by blaming China. The nation awaits the fallout from the 10-day rally in Sturgis S.D. where no mask policy is currently in place.

As one key Health official stated "There is no national strategy, no national leadership, and no urging for the public to act in unison, and carry out the measures together"

Not every country has made progress in containment and cases and deaths continue to rise. Surges continue in India, and the Philippines passed 100,000 reported cases, as well as new case spikes in Australia. In Melbourne, a curfew was put in effect from 8 p.m. to 5 a.m. with schools returning to home schooling and day care centers closed. India is recording over 50,000 cases per day and totals have surpassed 1.75 million infections. The month of July alone accounted for 1,1 million of those cases.

In Japan over 1,500 cases were reported, with the majority of the new cases, people in their 20's and 30's indicating the younger generation was letting its guard down.

In the U.S. too many groups and individuals are reluctant to abide by direction and refuse to wear masks. The annual event in Sturgis S.D. for example, went on as scheduled with over ½ million bikers converging on this small town, the majority without masks. As they return to their home base, the probability is they will carry back the virus and new outbreaks will surface.

As most countries struggle with the state of the pandemic, New Zealand is reaping the benefits of early aggressive decisions. They have passed 100 days with only a handful of infections from people returning from other countries, and then placed immediately in quarantine. Bars are open, soccer matches have stands filled with spectators. They made the decision in March to totally lock down the country. It paid in big benefits. The virus never got a chance to develop.

August 2020

All States in the U.S. move into August fac-ing School return decisions. Do they open? Do they partially open? home school only? Or delay? At one School in Atlanta, a child became infected after the first day of classes which made National news. Most schools are attempting to create a hybrid system to have half in classes on different days, to assist in the distancing requirement. Each State in the U.S. is developing a plan for their students. Decisions are being made for not only the elementary level students, but colleges and trade schools. In Minnesota, the school districts were given choices based on infection rates in their district area. In the individual districts, total acceptance and compliance was a major question as the teaching professionals remained concerned, and many parents had indicated their children would not return, forcing online schooling to remain an option. Transportation became an issue as busing was needed, and those vehicles plus the vehicles of parents who elected to drive their students, created traffic issues around the school properties every morning and afternoon. Additional staff was needed in schools for cleaning and monitoring halls, bathrooms, and lunchrooms. Older school facilities will need to review air replacement and square footage to meet COVID regulations. Some city systems have elected to maintain remote learning, as the return to classrooms is not feasible. As a secondary dilemma, fall and winter sports are under pressure to be delayed until spring. The Pro sports have revised their seasons and schedules, and will reopen with no fans and or limited fans at the games. The NFL has cancelled preseason, Baseball has a reduced schedule without fans, and Hockey is resuming in July on a playoff format for the Stanley cup. All sports teams have recorded infected players and staff, and many remain or are entering quarantine. Many conferences like the Big-10 have cancelled the fall season for 2020.

While the Pandemic continues to run a course far from being under control, vaccine development continues to reportedly make some progress here in the U.S, and countries around the world. The biggest test in the U.S. got underway in August with 30,000 volunteers receiving shots on a program from the National Institute of Health. Moderna and Pfizer are also preparing to begin testing and are recruiting another 30,000 volunteers. Both of the current studies will enroll about 30,000 healthy people at around 89 different sites around the country this summer. Half will receive two shots of the vaccine 28 days apart, and half will receive a saltwater placebo. Neither the volunteers or the medical staff will know who is getting which of the two injections.

Several other vaccines made by China and by Britain's Oxford University began smaller final stage trials in Brazil, and other hard-hit countries earlier this month. The U.S. requires its own tests of vaccines for approval be conducted in this country. The Government funded projects will roll out a new study each month requiring 30,000 participants. A U.S. study of the Oxford shot is to begin in August, a Johnson and Johnson trial in September, and a Novavax trial in October. Currently over 150,000 people have applied on-line. Moderna has indicated they would be able to deliver 500 million doses this year with possibly up to 1 billion per year in 2021. The company did receive $1Billion in grants from the Federal Government, but has indicated it intends to make a profit on the sale of the vaccine, stating only it will be priced responsibly.

While nations work endlessly to discover and test vaccines, Russia announces they have approved and have begun to inoculate Russian citizens. The International Health community views this decision with skepticism, as the vaccine has only been tested in dozens of people and not for an extended period of time. Putin contends it has proven efficient and it forms a stable immunity. To support this release, he had one of his daughters inoculated. Scientists are concerned that to proceed without Phase 3 testing could backfire, with this apparent rush to begin massive injections without prolonged testing. By comparison, vaccines entering the final stage-testing in the U.S requires studies of multiple 30,000 people testing. Two such testing programs are underway with three more to begin before fall 2020. The vaccine developed in Russia, uses a different virus, the common cold adenovirus, that's been modified to carry genes for the "spike" protein that coats the coronavirus to recognize if a real COVID-19 infection comes along. It is a similar technology that's being developed by one of China labs and also Britain's Oxford University and AstraZeneca. Russia has indicated they intend to start advanced trials by August 15th in in the United Arab Emirates, Saudi Arabia and the Philippines, involving several thousand people. The WHO is in contact with the Russian scientists hoping to review their study data.

In early March as the virus made its way worldwide, and thousands of people were stranded on Cruise ships with other infected passengers and the ship's crew, many moored at sea as countries were reluctant to dock the ships, disembark the passengers who could be infected. Some remained at sea for weeks without a place to dock and on some occasions released to other ships at sea. Infected and sick passengers, needed hospitalization. The Navy docked one of their hospital ships for transfer and care of patients at sea.

Cities were not allowing ships to dock and at one point the Panama Canal refused passage of cruise ships. When the ships eventually were allowed to dock, the passengers in U.S. ports were housed in quarantine for 14 days before they were allowed to return home. Other Countries imposed similar regulations for passengers disembarking at their home ports.

While the passengers on these ships returned to their homes eventually, not all Cruise ship workers shared the same fate. August 1st it was reported over 12,000 workers remained on board 57 cruise ships either docked or moored at sea in U.S. waters They are caught in the middle of no ships being used in a cruise, and cruise ship companies needing a crew to maintain these vessels. While some are being paid on a regular basis, others are working at less pay and some have filed actions for stranded at sea without pay. They are forced to live on board for months after they were supposed to return home, with nothing to do. They have lived in this situation for 5 months.

By early August, the virus had infected over 20 million people worldwide. The real number is probably much higher due to reporting issues in many countries, and many unrecognized and/or mis-diagnosed. The cases of the infected took 6 months to reach the 10 million case level, and only 6 weeks more, to double to the current 20 million case level. Half of the infected people are from three countries. The U.S. with over 5 million cases, followed by India and Brazil. Daily case infections reported in the U.S. remains over 54,000 per day, and 59,000 and 44,000 in India and Brazil. The U.S death rate is now at 163,000, and continues to amaze the worlds scientific community that with all the valued ingenuity and head start the U.S. had over Europe and Asia in preparation time, it has been mass confusion The U.S. has about 4% of the world's population and accounts for about 25% of the world's known coronavirus infections and 22% of the deaths.

The European community which had massive infections in Spring and stabilized in early summer, gave the countries an opportunity to relax the restrictions and take advantage of the peak vacation period. By late August however restrictions were re-imposed as flareups disrupted vacations in many countries. Even in chic resort areas nightclubs were again closed, fireworks were banned, and mask orders reimposed. Alcohol fueled street parties and large family gatherings have been cited as the source of new outbreaks in several European countries.

In France, the vacationing Britons scrambled to return home to avoid having to self-quarantine for 14 days following Briton's decision to reimpose travel restrictions on travel from France because of a resurgence of infections there. Ferries and trains were running out of space to accommodate the vacationers returning from France. The British Government said it imposed the quarantine requirement due to a 66% increase in infections on people returning from France. Tough new measures were also put in place in Spain, which recorded almost 50,000 new COVID cases in the last 14 days. France, Briton, Spain and Italy have recorded over 140,000 deaths. Italy is also facing a surge of new infections. Beaches faced new restrictions with no fireworks, no overnight access, and requiring masks be worn outdoors. On Friday 8/15 Italy recorded 574 new cases, the highest level since May 28th.

In the U.S. on August 20th more than 5.4 million cases have been confirmed with over 170,500 deaths. The States of NY with

32,000, Calif with 11,000 Texas with 10,000 and Florida with 9,000 are high death areas. Recent reported infections continue to rise, California who reported over 60,000 in the last 7 days, Texas 54,000, and Florida with 56,000 continue to be the high-risk areas of the U.S. The rates continue to rise at uncontrolled levels, mostly because the American public refuses to follow guidelines and use common sense. The U.S. is looked on world-wide as a base of people who have a lack of concern for others. Mask wearing, although a mandate is randomly followed at best, as is requirements of social distancing and crowd restrictions. The recent Sturgis Motorcycle Rally in Sturgis S.D. where over ½ million gathered for a week of wild partying has resulted in the beginning of new COVID infections in many states. States had 140 recorded infections by attendees in August, and that does not take into account the number of infections spread as a result of their involvement at the rally. South Dakota does not have a policy of wearing masks, so few attendees took the responsibility to protect themselves and others.

Minnesota has lower continued death and infection rates with most recent days recording deaths in the single digits. The death toll now stands at 1,800, with over 66,000 confirmed cases. Of those infected, 75% Of the deaths were residents of long-term care facilities. Minnesotans with the largest infected rates are in their 20's. but have a smaller number of deaths.

As August 2020 heads into its final days, the virus continues to infect hundreds of thousands world- wide and impacts every segment of individual lives. Schools at every level here in the U.S. are in limbo on starting dates and actual direction. Some states had restrictions by district on qualifications for openings. Could the district could fully reopen, partially reopen, or continue with virtual learning. Parents are struggling to decide a course of action for their family unit. If they decide not to enroll their child in the in the person program at school, and continue with remote virtual learning in their home, they are faced with hiring supervision in their home. As parents begin to return to the workplace in many areas, no longer is parent supervision available. Parents with partial classroom learning and partial in-home virtual learning are attempting to find supervision help, and the demand far exceeds the people available as home nannies.

Private schools in Minnesota for the most part have opted to open with full time classroom learning. State Law requires the Private sector be funded by district at the same rate as the public schools, and if the district has decided to maintain full or part remote learning for public schools, a variety of support services will not be available to the Private sector, such as busing, nursing, counseling, and other services. As August ended and September was about to begin, many school issues, at all school levels, remained in limbo across the U. S., and many Colleges delayed openings. As colleges did begin to open across the U.S, many outbreaks are begin-ning to surface as students begin to gather. Some colleges are reporting over 100 new infections almost daily, causing problems with opening classes.

By the end of August, a resurgence of COVID had begun in Spain recording 53,000 cases the last week in August. Other European countries, France, Belgium, Italy, and Germany are experiencing similar increases in infections as August comes to an end, but the progression in Spain is recording new infec-tions twice as fast as France, eight times the rate in Italy and Britain, and 10 times the pace in Germany. Spain was one of the hardest hit countries initially, with over 440,000 infected cases and 29,000 deaths. It had one of the most stringent lockdowns, which did check the spread, and then they enjoyed one of the most rapid re-openings of any of the European countries. The return of nightlife and group activities, beach enjoyment, the return of tourism, and the decision to return responsibility for combating the virus to local authorities after the national lockdown, has contributed to the Pandemics resurgence. The median age of sufferers has now dropped to 37 from 60. Greece has now suspended all flights from Greece to Spain in an effort to control the spread to their country

India recorded 78,761 new cases in one day the last Sunday of August, the largest single spike since the beginning of the virus. This happened just as India was beginning to ease restrictions to help their battered economy. India now has the fastest growing daily caseload of any country in the world, reporting more than 75,000 new cases per day for 4 straight days.

REPORTED CASES AND DEATHS AUGUST 31st 2020

COUNTRY	CASES	TOTAL DEATHS
World	25,595,000	855,000
USA	6,205,000	188,000
Brazil	3,910,000	121,400
India	3,700,000	65,500
Russia	955,400	17,200
Peru	648,000	29,000
South Africa	628,000	14,200
Columbia	608,000	19,400
Mexico	595,000	64,200
Spain	463,000	29,100
Chili	412,000	11,300

Some areas of the U.S showed some positive signs as September began, particularly in the Southeast Sunbelt, which had recorded more than 35,000 deaths the past two months. Florida's death rate has dropped to about 114 per day, from a high of 185 in early August. The Florida Governor announced he is easing some restrictions to allow visitors to Nursing Homes which had been banned for over 5 months. While some States had some positive results, others recorded different trends. Minnesota recorded over 20,400 new cases in August, the highest monthly total since the virus began. Other Midwest States recorded similar trends. Many factors are contributing to the trends, larger gatherings, like the fallout from the Sturgis rally, postponed weddings and funerals which are now being held, and a population movement away from home isolation.

In an attempt to begin a return to normalcy, South Carolina approved a plan for 8,000 people to attend a NASCAR event

SEPTEMBER 2020

As September begins, the activity on the vaccine approaches the final stages of testing. Several companies are beginning the final stages of testing, here in the U.S. and worldwide. Astra Zeneca an England based company will test over 30,000 people here in the U.S. from various racial, geographic and ethnic groups. Other companies are testing in Brazil, China, and Russia. The tests involve development of anti-bodies and virtually every other imaginable approach to containing this worldwide dilemma.

Beginning September 2020 changes continued and countries around the world struggled with school openings and controlling crowds. States and countries without mandates on wearing masks began to face growing infection rates. The Rally in Sturgis South Dakota which was unrestricted has been termed a Super Spreader. A model developed by a research company has determined the Rally could be linked to over 250,000 cases of infections in the period August 2nd to September 2nd. For the progression of the Pandemic, Sturgis is what could be described as the perfect storm. The State of South Dakota failed to develop restrictions, and the participants of the Rally represent the element of society that prides itself as a group without rules. It is projected the ultimate health costs of this Rally will be in the billions, to the American people.

The week following Labor Day is School beginning for most of the U.S. and distance learning became the route for many school districts. The worst thing that could possibly add to the dilemma, was a potential breakdown in the computer learning website, which provides the technology to the individual schools and students. Over 70 of the top 100 School systems with students from K-12, had major issues with failure of the websites, to either load or load slowly, and students unable to register.

As schools open here in Minnesota and Globally, various learning processes, have been established to meet local State and District needs. Many opening processes are on a temporary basis as the Pandemic begins to become controllable, adaptions can and will be made. Minnesota Department of Education released their breakdown and most other Sates probably duplicate this variance.

44% are using a combination mode.

23 % are offering full in person classes for all students who want it.

20 % have all grades on a part time schedule.

13 % are offering only distance learning at all grade levels.

The school re-openings and the variation of scheduling, puts parenting in a very difficult position. Day care centers are full, and due to distance requirements have reduced student count admittance. Students in homes with multiple students in distance learning, continue to have scheduling difficulties with computer time between family members.

Also, as the colleges reopen and students begin to move into student housing, parties, drinking, lack of masks, and social distancing has brought the 20's age group to record levels of infections.

As a concern to many, the Big Ten Football conference reversed its decision to cancel the 2020 season and agreed to a 12-game schedule to begin October 23rd – 24th.

By mid-September the WHO issued an appeal based on their analysis that the World's major powers were failing to fight the Pandemic together. They reported more than 300,000 new cases were reported in the past 24 hours globally, with India, United States, Argentina, Brazil and Spain recording the largest gains. The WHO has recorded more than 31 million infections and close to 1 million associated deaths. The WHO officials pointed out that the reported numbers tell only part of the story. Countries face major problems even with small numbers in many countries. Yemen for example with about 2,000 cases and 600 deaths, are involved in numerous regional power wars that involve regional control. In addition to the pandemic crisis, they are struggling an epidemic crisis, of lack of food, other diseases and a collapsing health system. Other countries face similar circumstances, which for many reasons are not factored into the Pandemic reporting.

The death toll in the U.S passed 200,00, the highest in the World. The number of deaths is equivalent to a 9/11 attack every day for 67 days. Deaths are continuing at over 770 per day and could double to over 400,000 by the end of the year, with colder weather setting in, and colleges and schools reopening. We are far from managing this crisis. The U. S, for the past 5 months, has led the world by far in sheer numbers, and infections with no sign of relief. With over 7 million cases of infections, and over 200,000 deaths. We have 5% of the World's population and 20% of the Worlds deaths. Brazil is number 2 with 137,000 deaths and India with 89.000

India while currently ranking 3rd in total infections and deaths has about 1 million fewer cases than the US. but is catching up fast. The total reported cases this past month has doubled from 3 million cases to over 6 million infected cases. India has aggressively pursued contract tracing to reduce the Pandemic expansion especially in outlying communities.

In hindsight the U. S. while totally prepared from the worlds perspective to manage a pandemic, failed at every level. Monitoring at airports was loose, travel bans came too late. Too late did health officials realize the virus could spread before symptoms appeared, rendering screening imperfect. The virus swept into nursing homes exploiting poor infection controls, and claimed over 78,000 lives. At the same time, gaps in leadership led to shortages of testing supplies, and warnings to ramp up production of masks were ignored, leaving states to compete for protective gear. The administration downplayed the threat and complained that too much testing was making the U.S. look bad, and turned it into a political issue. On April 10th the president predicted the U.S. wouldn't see 100,000 deaths in 2020. That milestone was reached on May 27th.

In the U.K as September was coming to a close, new restrictions were put in place as the Prime Minister appealed for a spirit of togetherness through the winter, as they recorded over 4,900 new cases, which was the highest daily total since early May, and four times higher than the total one month ago. The big change came in requiring Restaurants and Pubs to close at 10 P.M. Mask usage was also expanded. They assume the new restrictions would be in place for at least 6 months.

OCTOBER 2020

The WHO stated on October 6th that 1 in 10 people world-wide have probably been infected with the virus, more than 20 times the numbers being reported, and that a very difficult period lies ahead. The outbreaks vary by rural and regional areas, but the vast majority of the world remains at risk. Southeast Asia faced a surge in cases, as has Europe and the eastern Mediterranean, while the situations in Africa and the Western Pacific were more stable. The estimates from the WHO on numbers of infected cases would indicate 760 million people have been infected, far exceeding the 35 million now being reported. Concerns continue to exist between the WHO and the Chinese government on transparencies of data and the access being given to the mission's members. China continues to indicate they are transparent and responsive.

Evidence now shows the Chinese Government had evidence of this virus as early as December 12th with someone displaying symptoms, but the Wuhan Health authorities did not reveal the outbreak to the public until December 31st. Meanwhile the threat of the virus was downplayed by the Chinese Government, and in Wuhan, it was business as usual. In advance of the Chinese New Year January 18th large social gatherings took place with 40,000 or more at dinners sharing food and social life. Over 5 million people from Wuhan traveled throughout China in celebration and scores of people carried the virus. On January 14th the Wuhan health organization citing their research, stated that there was no clear evidence of human-to-human transmission. Days later on January 20th the Chinses regime admitted the virus was contagious. The first death confirmed as a COVID death took place on January 9th. The man worked at the Wuhan Food market where the virus reportedly was linked to the outbreak. On February 26th it was confirmed that the Chinese Government had three of their gene-sequencing companies working on a sequence of samples they received in December 2019. It wasn't until January 12th that the Chinese regime shared the announcement to the WHO to share with researchers around the world.

New data was beginning to show that college campuses have become massive threat outbreaks across the U.S. There were over 80,000 new infections recorded on 1,200 campuses as of early September. The additional threat is the chain reaction of the infections as they move back and forth to their home communities and family units, to more vulnerable people with whom they come in contact with. Testing in some of the southern states showed an increase in those in the 20 to 30 age group followed by an increase 9 days later, in the 40 to 59 age group, and another increase in the 60 plus age group 15 days later. The younger age group needs to understand the role they play in the transmission and expansion of the virus among the total population.

October brought a new reality to the COVID -19 virus here in the U.S. and worldwide. The President of the U.S and his wife and head of staff, were diagnosed positive with COVID virus and placed in quarantine. The President was placed at Walter Reed Hospital and underwent various treatments. The

President continues to downplay the virus, even while undergoing treatments and contradicts everything the health community shares. Others of the White House staff also tested positive for the virus. Some were his closest advisors

New cases the past seven days in Wisconsin has progressed to over 17,500 reported cases, compared to neighboring Minnesota with 7,200. Wisconsin became one of the worst hotspots in the nation the past few weeks ranking 3rd nationwide with the number of new cases being reported. The Governor on October 6th issued new orders limiting the size of groups allowed in indoor public gatherings which impacted Restaurants and Bars. The orders are in effect until November 6th. The order limits indoor gatherings to 25% of the building's capacity, while indoor spaces without a capacity limit will be limited to 10 people. Those violating the order will face A $500.00 fine. Reactions from the Restaurants and the bars has been massive and owners are totally upset with the decision. Lawsuits have been initiated against the mandate of wearing masks, but the judge ruled in his favor and the mandate continues. Wisconsin is among the nation worst COCID -19 areas and has 152,000 reported cases and record numbers of outbreaks and deaths reported by October 13, 2020. The new aggressive number of cases, hospitalizations and deaths are attributed to opening of schools and uncontrolled socialization in the college campuses, and a general fatigue of virus restrictions. The crisis really began in early September as students returned to school. At that time the number of infection cases was about 700 and two weeks later it doubled and by Mid October was close to 3,000. 625 cases were reported per 100,000 residents over the past week, the 4th highest in the nation. One week later the new cases report had risen to 3,861, a new case record beating 3,747, record from the day before. Clearly the infection rate is out of control, The Governors order to limit the capacity of patrons in bars and Restaurants, was struct down by a Judge responding to a lawsuit from the Tavern League in the State. Another lawsuit is in place to end the Statewide mandate for wearing masks. The Republican Legislature contends he is exceeding his authority and doesn't seem to care about the impact on human lives. Hospitalizations have exceeded 1,100 per day in Wisconsin.

The State has built a field hospital at the Wisconsin State fairground with a capacity of 530 beds, as the surge in hospitalizations will soon overwhelm the ability of hospitals to handle the influx the expanding virus. Other States have constructed similar facilities. Nationally about 30,000 coronavirus patients are now hospitalized.

By mid-October, in Minnesota the number of recorded infections has begun again to rise in long term care facilities, currently there are about 341 long term care facilities which are recording new cases, the highest rate since July. The increase in new infections appears to be spreading within the communities and brought back into care facilities. Roughly 38% of the new infections are from community infections with the 20's group leading the high rate of new infections, but the high rate of deaths continues to be individuals 60 and over, 69 % of the deaths are from the long-term facilities. While the rates in long term have increased, the Governor loosened restrictions on seating in Restaurants to 10, from previous 4 per table, or 6 from one household per table. The 10 is in effect for both a family group or a non-family group. Bar seating will continue to be restricted to 4 per table.

Worldwide there is little sign of relief and daily infections continue to increase dramatically. The U.S continues to lead the world in numbers of infected cases and deaths. The slow management by the Government led the States and health officials on the wrong path.

By Country Mid October

COUNTRY	1ST INFECTION	TOTAL CASES	DEATHS	7-DAY
USA	1/21/20	7,856,605	215,887	UP
INDIA	1/29/20	7,175,888	109,856	DOWN
BRAZIL	2/25/20	5,113,628	150,998	DOWN
RUSSIA	1/30/20	1,318,783	22,834	UP
ARGENTINA	3/2/20	917,0035	24,572	DOWN
COLUMBIA	3/5/20	924,098	28,141	UP
SPAIN	1/31/20	896,086	33,204	DOWN
FRANCE	1/23/20	798,257	32,982	UP
UK	1/30/20	637,708	43,108	UP
ITALY	1/30/20	365,467	36,246	UP

Trends around the world show many with a 7-day growth trend, unfortunately the U.S leads the world. The proportion of Americans dying from the virus, is the highest in the developed world. Early in the outbreak, the U.S. mortality rate from COVD-19 was lower than most other high infected countries, including the U.K., Spain and the Netherlands, but as spring turned to summer, the U.S. largely failed to advance public health and policy, at the same pace as in other countries that controlled the virus expansion to reduce death rates. If the U.S.

deaths after May 10th had occurred at the same pace as in Spain, the U.S. mortality rate would be 47% lower than current levels and a total of 93,247 less people dying.

The world by late October had progressed to massive rates of infection growth and uncontrolled attempts to control the progression. As the population in virtually every country became weary of the requirements of quarantine, lack of masks and lack of social distancing became the norm. Restaurants and bars were becoming packed, and became an open opportunity for the transmission of the virus. Little interest in maintaining control was in effect, and was not under control. The progression and handling of the virus in the U.S. was completely out of control.

Not only nationally with the Presidential candidates, but States struggled with demands by one party or the other. Lawsuits became the norm as Governors tried to impose sanctions. In virtually every state, actions were met with resistance and conflict emerged. To add to the struggle in the U.S. racial conflicts continued to surface and demonstrations turned to riots, looting, deaths and injury. Several states dealt with massive unrest, and use of the National Guard to calm the unrest. Not only the unrest developed major issues with law enforcement, but the crowds involved disregarded social distancing and the wearing of masks. With the election less than one week away and the attitude of not only President Trump, but his followers, the outcome of the election will be disputed for an extended period of time, and increased civil unrest no matter the outcome is a virtual certainty. The U.S. faces not only the continued uncontrolled expansion of the Pandemic, but the sporadic support levels of the American people. What worries the medical community and the disease scientists, is that people have let their guard down. It's gone from infection issues in the big cities to rural communities. States which did not require citizens to wear masks are now paying a terrible high price. States like North Dakota, where no mask mandate was in place, now leads the nation in infections per day with 770 per 100,000 people, and 24 daily deaths. The National coronavirus coordinator who has traveled to over 40 states found the situation in North Dakota the worst she had seen. People in grocery stores and Restaurants even in hotels disregarded social distancing, and had the least use of masks of any states. On October 19th the Mayor of Fargo North Dakota used his emergency powers and issued a mandatory mask order, the first of its kind in the State. Hours later, the Mayor on Minot issued a similar order. We were hoping we had escaped the COVID-19, now we're just like everybody else. It has hit us with a vengeance.

Other areas of the U.S faced crisis situations. In El Paso TX a border town, authorities instructed people to stay home for two weeks and imposed a 10 p.m. to 5 a.m. curfew as hospitals had become overwhelmed. On October 25th, 853 cases were recorded in the county, versus 786 a day earlier overwhelming the hospitals. Part of the civic center began being used to house patients that the hospitals were unable to handle. The state already overwhelmed, is providing medical assistance to El Paso to deal with the rise in hospitalized cases in addition to many other cities.

In Idaho where large numbers of residents have resisted wearing masks, the Governor ordered a return to some restrictions as case rates put a strain on Hospitals. Idaho's positivity test rate is the fourth worst in the nation. Children requiring hospitalization are traveling 125 miles away, and elective surgeries are being postponed. A similar situation is unfolding in Oklahoma where COVID records are consistently being broken, and bed space is running out, coupled with a growing shortage of nursing staff.

In Florida, one of the hardest hit states, they made the decision to fully reopen bars and restaurants despite the fact that over 10% of the residents are testing positive according to a recent 7 day rolling forecast. The WHO had set a benchmark of 5% before reopening retail establishments. The Pandemic has killed Floridians of a rate of 65.8 per 100,000 with only 10 states having a higher death percentage. Dr. Fauci says this is very concerning and lacks common sense. Many other States that have reduced restrictions are suffering the consequences.

The U.S. the opening of schools in September continues to be a political nightmare. Many parents wanted full time reopening of schools, while many more, feared the impact of exposure to students would ultimately impact families and the total community. The State health authorities in many states, established guidelines for the State school Districts, many based on the percentage of infections in the immediate community. All states face difficult issues regarding distance learning, classroom learning, or a hybrid of some sort, and split schedules for students. While the impact of these issues is difficult for students and families, it's a compounded problem for teachers, staff and administration. Athletic participation became a hot issue as parents and student athletes were not prepared to eliminate fall sporting events, and eventually schedules were improvised for a limited number of games, and elimination in many cases of playoffs. Parents naturally made these decisions difficult, as they had difficulty looking at the exposure brought by these activities. This is true at the High School level, the college level and the professional level. Currently games are held at all levels minus fans, but games are being frequently cancelled as players are tested positive.

Worldwide, the virus progression continues at record levels as the month of October nears an end, and the infection and death rates are skyrocketing virtually everywhere. In Poland which had very low rates of infection in the Spring, announced its President Andrzej Duda, had tested positive but was feeling well under quarantine. The U.K. much like the U.S. is struggling with management of the virus as the political environment continues to impact decision making. Two regions in the U.K. chose to impose higher restrictions than the prime Minister requested. In Northern Ireland, they announced schools would close for two weeks, and pubs and Restaurants for four weeks, to slow the spread of the virus. Wales announced it would close visitation from other hot spots of the U.K. In Liverpool England, which has had one of the highest levels of infections, when the new tough restrictions were announced, people swarmed the streets, as bars were closing amid fears they may not reopen until spring.

Britain currently has massive progression. Northern Ireland has recorded 1,156 cases, per 100,000 people, compared to 995 in Wales, 960 in England and 755 in Scotland. In France the French Prime Minister announced a vast extension of the nightly curfew, stating the 2nd wave is here. A curfew had been imposed the prior week including Paris and the suburbs, and this announcement impacted 38 more regions starting Friday October 29th This is likely to last for six weeks or more. This means that 46 million of the country's 67 million will be under a 9 p.m. to 6 a.m. curfew which prohibits them from being out during those hours, except for limited reasons, Hours later the Health Department reported a record 41,600 new virus cases a new daily high. France is nearing 1 million reported cases of the virus.

There is little indication in Moscow that Russia is being swept up by a resurgence of the coronavirus. Bars and Restaurants in the city are packed, and little evidence of anyone other than the workers wearing masks, People are crowded together and disregard protective measures. The outbreak in October is setting new highs, breaking the record highs in the spring before a lockdown was put in place. On the 20th of October they reported aver 15,000 new infections the highest spike in the pandemic thus far. The spring lockdown hurt the economy, and drove Putin's approval to new lows. It's said people have come to an end of their tolerance of the lockdown measures, and it would be hugely unpopular if imposed again.

Spain, buckling under the resurgence of infections in Europe, declared a national state of emergency that includes an overnight curfew in hopes of not repeating the near collapse of the country's hospitals earlier. No free movements on the streets between 11 p.m. and 6 a.m. The curfew takes place November 1st and will likely last for 6 months. We are immersed in the 2nd wave and the situation is extreme according to the country's health officials. Spain became the first European Country to exceed 1 million reported cases. Elsewhere around the world, a new wave of lockdowns and restrictions swept across Europe. France, Germany, Italy, Greece, Switzerland, Bulgaria, as well as others, had imposed expanded lockdowns. As countries became overpowered by the 2nd wave. Italy recorded its highest daily total of over 25,000 cases, and Germany with over 15,000. In England the case total exceeded 1 million, and Prime Minister Johnson himself a COVD survivor announced a month-long lockdown, stating unless aggressive action was taken, the hospitals would be overwhelmed in weeks. The new restrictions impact bars and Restaurants which will be closed for in person dining, and can only offer take out service. Non-essential shops are to be closed. People will only be able to leave home for a short list of reasons. Unlike the earlier lockdown mandate, schools, Universities, Manufacturing plants and construction sites, will remain open. The ruling requires the approval of Parliament which will vote on the matter on Wednesday November 4th. One Senior Parliament Official indicated the lockdown could last considerably longer if the daily rates continue to climb.

MID OCTOBER CS/DEATHS BY COUNTRY, WITH MONTH END COMPARISON.

Date Of 1st Infection		Mid Month		End of Month		
		CASES	DEATHS	CASES	DEATHS	PER 1 MIL
USA	1/21/20	7,856,605	215,887	9,430,204	236,235	712
INDIA	1/29/20	7,175,888	109,856	8,214,596	122,475	88
BRAZIL	2/25/20	5,113,628	150,998	5,535,605	159,902	750
RUSSIA	1/30/20	1,318,783	22,834	1,636,781	28,235	193
ARGENTINA	3/2/20	917,035	24,572	1,166,944	31,002	684
COLUMBIA	3/5/20	924,098	31,314	1,074,184	31,314	613
SPAIN	1/31/20	896,086	33,204	1,264,517	35,87	767
FRANCE	1/23/20	798,257	32,982	1,367,625	36,788	563
UK	1/30/20	637,708	43,108	1,034,914	46,717	687
ITALY	1/30/20	365,467	36,246	679,428	38,618	163

Worldwide Total   **46,642,965   1,203,256   154**

November 2020

B efore the end of the first week of November 2020, Europe was making a major effort to halt the 2nd wave, now rampant throughout the European countries. England had announced they would begin a 2nd lockdown beginning on Friday, and it was unanimously approved by parliament on the 4th of November. The Italian Government announced on Wednesday they will lock down a significant portion of their country.

Heading into November, the surge of new infections was sweeping across the U. S. and virtually every country in the World. In the U.S. total confirmed cases exceeded 9 million cases. The number of new cases reported daily is on the rise in 47 states. The new case numbers eclipse the warning increases set in place last spring. Over the past two weeks the daily infection total of over 76,000 cases far surpasses the daily average of 54,000 in mid-October, with little relief in sight. The main problem in the U.S. is the total lack of personal responsibility. Governors and or Legislatures continue to play politics with lock downs, masks and/or restrictions. It would appear many politicians choose not to protect the citizens, choosing instead to cater to the political party system demands. The action of Governors and Legislatures reflect the way that politics, and the personal beliefs of a significant sector of the population have become entangled with supposedly nonpartisan matters of public health. It's become a blame game from the national to the local level. In virtually every other country of the World, leaders have made difficult decisions on lockdowns, crowd control and mask mandates, while the U. S. leaves its people at risk. In the U.S. transmission control measures were announced March 15th. A study has confirmed that social distancing and control measures put in place a week earlier, could have led to 600,000 fewer cases, and possibly 32,000 deaths

Election day is November 3rd and it is presumed, the outcome will present, whoever wins, a devastating situation for 1 year, possibly more. When election day in the U.S. had come and gone, Biden has the lead in enough states to claim victory. The country has been focused on the election process, and little concern appears to focused against the pandemic which is setting National daily records, in virtually every states. On November 6th, the U.S. surpassed 120,000 cases for the 2nd day in a row. In addition, 20 states have set a record day during the month of November. As the second week of November begins, not only has the U.S. President totally ignored the dramatic increase in the pandemic, but refuses to concede he lost the election. At his election parties and gatherings, masks were not expected to be worn, and were not, nor was social distancing observed, and now his immediate staff is facing the consequences. His chief of Staff on November 6th was tested as Positive and a follow up of at least 5 others were also diagnosed. No further announcements are being allowed regarding the infections of his personal staff. His infected staff, now join days after the election, over 10 million other infected American's citizens and deaths approaching 240,000 people.

The total U.S. continues to set record numbers with the daily new confirmed cases, surging 45% in the past two weeks, to a record 7-day average of 87,000 new cases, and deaths have increased 15% to an average of 850 people losing their life daily. On November

6th, 111,000 new cases were recorded in the U.S. in one day The Midwest has become a hotspot, with North Dakota, South Dakota, Iowa, and Wisconsin among the leading areas being infected. North and South Dakota have the nation's worst rate of deaths in the U.S. over the past 30 days. These states were reluctant to impose any restrictions on the people in the state, on masks, size of group activity, and now face a situation which is becoming uncontrollable. The Medical community is rapidly facing insurmountable problems with available space and health care workers. Rural Medical care is pushed beyond its ability to admit, and staff the limited number of hospitals. They are being transported to the larger cities, which puts a huge strain on not only the available health care in the larger cities, but the family's ability to support those infected, hospitalized away from their home cities.

North Dakota reported 309 people died in the last 30 days, more than all other periods combined. They shot to the top of the nation in deaths per capita in the last 30 days, with 41. South Dakota reported 252 deaths the past 30 days a 98% increase, and deaths of 29 per 100,000. Both of the States have basically ignored any restrictions beginning with the Sturgis Motorcycle rally in Sturgis South Dakota, in August which drew over 500,000 people. Few were wearing masks and social distancing was nonexistent. This was the beginning of a massive increase in infections. Both of the Governors refused to issue any mask mandate, leaving it up to the individuals. Obviously, this hasn't been successful.

On a recent tour while in Bismarck, N.D, Dr. Brix, the White House Coronavirus coordinator shook her head at what she saw, saying she saw less use of masks than anywhere she had been. The Governors of both States have made it clear they will not issue mask mandates. Both are Republicans and strongly follow the direction Of Trump.

Wisconsin had more than 6,000 cases in one day as the virus continues to rage across the state. The actions by the Governor to order limits on how many people can gather in bars and restaurants was found by an appeals court as unenforceable and invalid on November 6ᵗʰ as 6,141 new cases were recorded in the state, and 62 more deaths. The Republican legislature has sought to block every effort by the Governor to impose control efforts. Currently Wisconsin has recorded 99.3 new cases per 100,000 people the last seven days. This number continues to grow. One week prior the rate was 80.3.

In virtually every state in the U.S. officials struggle with school programs not only by state, but attempting to manage the schools by district. Many Districts have attempted classroom learning in some form of a hybrid, but as the progression on the disease escalates, more and more remote learning becomes the norm.

The virus has had a major impact in nursing care facilities, with both the residents and the care workers. Infections have increased fourfold from May, to the beginning of November. National weekly reported infections of residents of 1,083, has risen to 4,274, with death rates more than doubling from 318 to 699. Equally concerning was the rate of staff infections in nursing facilities increasing from 855 per week in May, to over 4,000, by November. The Nursing and long-term care facilities account for 1% of the U.S. population, but account for 40% of the COVIC-19 deaths. The consensus is the Nursing facilities bear some responsibility, as many do not comply with basic infection controls. A study was done involving 20 states and one in 6, were not maintaining the testing records of staff, one in four had shortage of staffing personnel, and one in four reported shortages in protective supplies, such as masks and gowns. As hospitalization space becomes more critical, the nursing home population needs to find a way of controlling their population.

Many States are revising their pandemic restrictions, but with the current president refusing to concede the election, his followers blindly follow his refusal to wear masks and avoid crowded areas. In States with Republican Governors mandates are non-existent. In both of the Dakotas, which are recording record numbers of infections, the Governors still refuse to invoke controls, despite demands by the public.

While the U.S. numbers are setting record infections and deaths, the worldwide community is recording its highest numbers to date. In France, a new record was reached November 6th where in a 24-hour period, new cases surpassed 60,000 cases for the 2nd day in a row. Russia also recorded its highest daily number since the virus began, reporting 20,582 new cases and over 29.000 deaths. Russia has seen a surge in daily cases throughout October setting daily records almost every day. The Russian Health Minister imposed a nationwide mask mandate requiring people to wear masks in public places, on public transportation, and in parking lots and elevators. President Putin has visions of beginning mass vaccinations by the end of the year. Two vaccines have been registered for domestic use ahead of large-scale Phase 3 trials.

In Germany in November, a new daily record of 20,000 cases was set in a single day. The number of people requiring intensive care in Germany has doubled in the last 10 days.

Italy reported 35,505 new cases on November 5th and 445 deaths bringing its case total to 825,000 cases and over 40,000 deaths.

In the U.K, they recorded, the 2nd highest daily jump in COVID cases the day before England entered a second lockdown.

In India, schools reopened for students in Grades 9 and 10 after 8 months of closure due to the Pandemic. As the staff and students were tested with classes opening, 829 teachers and 575 students tested positive with the COVID infection. Despite the high rate of infections schools will remain open.

In Portugal, a curfew was imposed to slow the dramatic new case infection rates, which effects 70% of the Nation's population. On weeknights a curfew is in effect from 11:00 P.M. to 5 A.M. On weekends it's more restrictive, as you can only be out in the morning until 1 P.M. unless buying essentials at Grocery stores or making other essential purchases. This curfew is in effect for two weeks and will be evaluated after that period.

Hungary announced its strictest curfew 8 p.m. to 5 a.m. All businesses must close by 7 p.m.

Deaths continue at a record pace with very little let up in sight in virtually every part of the world.

WORLDWIDE DEATHS   FEBRUARY -NOVEMBER 2020

MONTHLY	TOTAL REPORTED DEATHS	REPORTED DAILY
FEBRUARY	304	45
MARCH	3,050	73
APRIL	50,598	5,349
MAY	244,904	5.882
JUNE	389,399	3,237
JULY	531.143	4,965
AUGUST	699,491	5716
SEPTEMBER	876,477	5,978
OCTOBER	1,031,471	5,623
NOVEMBER	1,207,648	5,481

CORONAVIRUS
VACCINE UPDATE

C urrently 4 companies are at the late stage of testing for a vaccine. Two companies, Astra Zeneca and Johnson and Johnson recently halted trials, due to reactions from participants in their trials, but have now been cleared by the Federal Health regulators to resume trials. Astra Zeneca had been under a six week pause to evaluate neurological issues from two participants in their trials. It was determined the reactions by these two individuals were not related to the trials and approval was given to resume testing.

4 major coronavirus vaccines are now being developed for infection control in the U. S. and have entered Phase 3 clinical trials. The companies involved in development are J& J, Astra Zeneca and the University of Oxford, BioNTech and Pfizer, and Moderna.

There are basically three categories of Vaccines that are moving froward. There are Protein Vaccines, Nucleic acid vaccines, and vital vectors. There would appear to be pluses and minuses to each type of vaccine.

Astra Zeneca and J&J vaccines are viral-vector, while Moderna, and Pfizer's are messenger RNA vaccines. An RNA vaccine has never been approved by the Food and Drug

Administration, while only one approved Viral-vector vaccine, which was Merck and Co. Ebola vaccine, which was approved last December.

Protein based vaccines are similar to the flu shot, and while effective, it requires subsequent dosages. J&J has a single-dose vaccine in test in Ireland, and a test involving a two-dosage trial. Another factor being researched is refrigeration of the vaccines during and after transport. Temperature requirements to maintain quality and effectiveness has been a challenging issue for vaccination programs. Currently, the success rate expected is in the 50% area with long term goals of 60 to 70 % to aid long term containment of the virus. Most experts do not foresee the first generation of COVID-19 vaccines to reach this goal.

The current timelines by the Drug Companies are late-stage development by the end of the year for J&J. Moderna expects Phase three readout by late November or December, and BioNTech and Pfizer by the end of October. Another late comer to the development is Novavax which is beginning late-stage testing in England and expects to begin new trials in the U.S. in coming months. 11 companies worldwide have now reached some final level of development of a vaccine.

As November progresses, Russia announces its Coronavirus Vaccine, Sputnik V, shows over 90% efficiency in test bases of 40,000 volunteers. Russia in August became the first country to approve a Covid-19 vaccine despite skepticism in the west over the speed of their development, and those trials were still ongoing. Since those trials, they have developed a second vaccine, and say a third could be in the making. Russia has also begun to market the Sputnik V vaccine to other countries including Brazil, India, Mexico and Egypt. Russia expects to begin a massive vaccination campaign in the coming weeks. The vaccine is to be given in two doses.

Meanwhile Pfizer and partner BioNTech indicate their vaccine has proven over 90% effective and will immediately take the lead in the all-out global race. They are now on track to seek emergency approval before the end of the year, and be able to produce limited initial dosages. The announcement by Pfizer was met with great enthusiasm by many in the scientific community, and with distain by Trump who contends the announcement was held until after the election in an effort not to give him credit. Pfizer contends it is not moved by politics, rather moved at the speed of science. Pfizer initially opted not to join the Trump Warp speed funding program instead investing its own money in the development. But in July the Company signed an agreement with the Government, to supply 100 million doses, assuming it would be cleared by the FDA. The FDA is currently reviewing the testing results from Pfizer.

Pfizer would begin production and distribution hopefully before the end of 2020, and have 30 to 40 million doses available by years end. This however would accommodate only 15 to 20 million people as two doses are required. The vaccine has been tested on people over 65, but in September included those as young as 16. Tests are now underway for as young as 12. One issue that appears to be confusing, is that the Pfizer BioNTech is a partnership, and BioNTech is a British Company. Reports circulating from British authorities is they will have the vaccine around Christmas, and will begin vaccinating by year end. It would appear that the production of this vaccine will involve a worldwide distribution, while we appear to be assuming this great new vaccine will be an American solution. There is however great optimism on the other pharmaceutical companies who have progressed to stage three trials. As these companies get approvals to begin production, it would be a great boom to the world Health community.

As the success of the Pfizer virus development gains legs, an announcement by Moderna that its vaccine has a 94.5% effective rate according to recent testing and they have applied for emergency approval. This means we have two companies that have vaccines with a hope for distribution, and ultimate slowdown of the virus explosion which is attacking the U.S. and the worldwide community. The announcements by Pfizer brought optimistic response from the 10 other vaccines now in different levels of trial. The success of other manufacturers is being met with great enthusiasm as Pfizer, and BioNTech cannot meet the needs of the total Global Pandemic.

CONTINUED U.S. PANDEMIC LACK OF DIRECTION.

By November 15th, Biden has clearly won the U.S. election and is now recording over 300 electoral votes with 270 needed for confirmation, as U.S. President. Trump continues the needless dialog in sighting people to protest, and no firm direction on this pandemic, which continues to take needless lives. Clearly it is time to take responsibility, admit your defeat and give direction to the professionals who can help get this under control. The U.S. is making itself vulnerable to the worldwide community.

On November 1st the U.S. was reporting 9,514,333 cases and 236,924 deaths. Ten days later, 1 million more were infected, and less than 1 week later on the 15th of November 2020, the numbers had skyrocketed to 11,398,400 cases, with 156,000 in one day. Total deaths were 251,557, with an increase of 301 new deaths in the last day. This was the 11th day in a row with more than 100,000 new confirmed cases. Ten states set daily records on the same day, and 29 states added more cases than any other week since the beginning of the pandemic. More than 1,200 deaths were recorded in one day, pushing the daily average to 1,120, a 38% increase from the averages two weeks prior. It's estimated that 2.2 million Americans have lost someone close to them, either as a family member, or close friend or associate. Fears are this could escalate to the 1918 Influenza pandemic that cost 50 million people worldwide their lives. During that pandemic, people were dying in the streets, as there was no place for their care. The medical community then, and could become now, so overwhelmed that the system literally breaks apart. Clearly the pandemic in this country is totally out of control. The U.S. has no unified controls which has been the basis for progress against the virus in other countries of the world. Every State has developed its own set of controls and or restrictions, with little or no coordination on what surrounding/ adjoining states have set in place. What has developed is 50 individual populated areas with controls independent of others, and complete lack of programs which support each other.

States which dug their feet in the sand as the virus gained foothold are suffering the consequences as the current phase of infections skyrockets. States like North Dakota with a Republican governor who refused to impose any restrictions or mandates, now has a pandemic out of control. He is taking what he called a business-friendly approach that puts the responsibility for slowing the virus on individuals, rather than Government mandates, so as to protect both the individual and their livelihood. His strategy has taken his state to the leadership of the country in rates of infections and deaths, and has pushed the states medical facilities beyond its breaking point. In addition to Hospitals being beyond capacity, health care workers are non-existent, as huge numbers were infected and are quarantined. Some are now back working as recovering infected workers, under a program approved by the CDC which permits these workers to return to work under extreme conditions. On November 14th, the Governor relented and imposed a mask mandate statewide.

The state of South Dakota appears to be a maverick in the massive movement to control the growth of the virus. The Governor on November 17th refused to issue a mandate on masks, or any additional restrictions for the residents. They like North Dakota are leading the nation on infected cases, and deaths per 100,000 residents both which continue to grow.

The impact of the dramatic explosion in case infection numbers and deaths, dramatically effects every facet of local government and community life. New restrictions imposed now in most states on lockdowns, closures, and the entire education system, have people worn out from a lifestyle change, which for many is far too difficult to handle. Schools for the most part have moved to distance learning, K – 12 and college levels. As the distance learning is implemented, the added difficulty for families to deal with this adjustment becomes an insurmountable challenge. Parents are now unable to leave while their children are in the distance learning, if they are not old enough to be left alone. Child care centers are overwhelmed, with little or no space available. A parent or parents who are in the healthcare system, have little or no option of staying home to supervise family students, and without family members to sit in, are stressed beyond belief with little relief or end in sight. These type situations complicate an already impossible family environment, across the entire nation and every single State. The approaching Thanksgiving Holiday, followed by Christmas, has the health care community in a very nervous state. Families are being urged to abstain from family gatherings, as bringing groups together who have had exposures from numerous sources, will do nothing but expand an already out of control disease progression.

In the U.S. by November 19th hospitalizations have increased daily for the past 24 days, and reached new heights the past 9 day. Deaths topped the quarter million mark in the U.S. as the infection continues to surge across the country. The totals come after at least 1,923 people died from the COVID virus on November 18th and 172,391 new case infections were recorded.

By the 22nd of November, worldwide infections reached 59,000,000 cases, with 484,240 cases in the last 24 Hrs. Total deaths reached 1,393,190 with 7,732 the last 24 Hrs. The U.S. continues to exceed all countries in the world, by unimaginable levels of 12,572,915 total reported case infections, 132,569 new and 262,691 deaths, 861 new in the last 24 hrs. Clearly the Pandemic is out of control, and the political standoff in this country places every American and every American family at risk. The U.S. residences are expected to forgo the family Thanksgiving celebration, and the Christmas celebrations everyone looks forward to. The American people are in limbo. Unfortunately, the delegation representing people of the U.S in congress, are really not representing the American people, for some reason are bowing to power sources, who do not share the values of the people they represent.

While most states in the U.S. have gone to distance learning, having tried hybrids of various variations, the increase in positive testing has brought local and state government to decisions of implementing distance learning in virtually every state. While the U.S. moves to distance learning, Europe and Foreign countries have moved in the opposite direction, and opened up classroom education, but with increased restrictions on masks, social distancing, one-way hallways, and enforced behavior of students. The European and non-U.S. countries have the advantage of much better control of the behavior, of not only the student base, but the population in general. Our political dilemma in the handling of the Pandemic and lack of effective direction has given people the feeling that they are exempt from the restrictions, and that they do not apply to them. But a lack of compliance impacts every age group. When the parents will not comply, how can we expect the student base to be committed to comply. We are at a breaking point, as stated by health care experts and the health Care community.

In the US Midwest states, where some States appeared to have some control, things have dramatically changed. States like North and South Dakota which had refused to comply with restrictions, are now paying a terrible price with record infections and deaths increasing on a daily basis. Minnesota which had implemented restrictions on residents early in the spring, set new restrictions to expire on December 17th for bars and restaurants, as well as other business units, like health clubs and social gatherings. Records are exceeded daily on infections and deaths. Most recently on November 18th and 19th the daily deaths reached 67 and 76. Of the recorded deaths, long term care facilities continue to be the hardest hit with approximately 70 % of the deaths originating in those facilities. In Wisconsin, every day sets new records, and the state wide mandate on masks, will now extend into January 2021. Hospitals are at the breaking point with no relief is in sight. 8,000 new cases were added on November 18th bringing the total to 331,837 since the pandemic started. The seven-day average for new cases is 6,653, up from 1,563 two months ago. 48 of the 50 States, are recording daily case and death increases. Virtually every State has imposed restrictions to slow the expansion of the virus with varying degrees of success mainly dependent upon compliance of the local residents. Most have attempted to set in motion, actions to reduce what could be a devastating upcoming holiday period. Many states have closed all restaurants and bars and restricted other business activity. While not popular with many elements of the public, the medical community cannot keep up with the uncontrolled expansion and the demands on hospitals. The U. S. faces the biggest challenge in its history and the political standoff continues to complicate the entire control of the disease. The current President of the U.S. refuses to concede his loss to Joe Biden, and in his, egotistical refusal, has completely impacted the country's ability to address the management of the pandemic. The progress of the approval of the vaccines and data in the CDC, needs to be shared, as is the tradition in the transfer of power in every election. That is being entirely ignored and the President's actions continue to make it virtually impossible to manage any type of transition which would help move the pandemic to a more manageable level.

The virus has impacted all segments of the worldwide community. The WHO headquarters in Geneva Switzerland recorded 65 positive virus confirmations among their staff. The mayo clinic in Minnesota, reports over 900 of their staff have been infected to date. The infection activity at the Mayo has been traced to community transmissions rather than staff transmissions.

Early in the pandemic many passengers on Cruise ships were stranded as worldwide ports refused to grant permission to dock, as a large number of people on some ships, had been confirmed positive and the ports were not prepared to handle the infected people, or place the other passengers in quarantine for the required period as dictated by Country officials of the ports. Many passengers remained at sea, for up to two weeks confined to their cabins with meals left by their door. If you were fortunate enough to have an outside room with a balcony, the quarantine was livable, but if you were in an inside room with no windows or exposure to the outside, it became a nightmare. While ultimately the passengers all were allowed to disembark, the cruise ship companies, as the pandemic developed, basically ceased operations, are not operating to any extent. While virtually all cruise lines have harbored the majority of their ships, a few have sailed. Mid-November, a 7-day cruise from Barbados on the Sea Dream 1, two passengers had tested positive, even after two tests prior to sailing were required, and every passenger was confirmed negative. Since the initial discovery, 6 additional passengers have tested positive, and the ship had anchored off Bridgetown as more tests were conducted. All of the 53 passengers are confined to their rooms. Clearly every segment of society and life is impacted by the progression of this disease.

As the U.S heads into the week of Thanksgiving, which is traditionally a week of celebration with families, gatherings will be unlike any in history, with restrictions and strong requests by Government and the health community, to eliminate or drastically reduce the numbers of people involved in multi-family events. While Thanksgiving week has typically involved extensive travel for a large part of our population, the air travel is at the lowest level ever recorded. The risk associated with family and celebration gatherings, has brought massive rates of infections within the last few weeks with weddings and other gatherings. One wedding in Tulsa Oklahoma resulted in 85 infected participants, and an unknown number of residual infected people from attendance at the event. Many families have decided to do dinner with only the immediate family, in their home. Restaurants throughout the country are restricted from in unit dining, and will only do take-out and deliveries, to accommodate their customers. Mask mandates are in place in virtually every state. In Los Angeles, restaurants and bars are completely closed beginning November 24th. In Las Vegas, casinos are restricted to 25 % occupancy for the next four weeks. Many bars and restaurants have added new restrictions. Here in Minnesota, bars and restaurants are closed, with the exception of take out, and curbside for the next three weeks. All athletic activity is suspended, and closures of businesses, includes gyms and health clubs. Churches can remain open, but with severe restrictions on occupancy and protective measures in place. Nearby Wisconsin has implemented upgraded restrictions with a mask mandate and other protective mandates. Virtually every state in the U.S. and every foreign country has made new restrictions on behavior, travel, and social activity, with lock-downs from mostly 10 P.M. until early morning. Gatherings and limits of gatherings, are being restricted virtually world-wide. Never before in the history of the world have this many people, been faced with anything of the magnitude, for this long of a period of time and with an unknown future.

The situation is beyond critical worldwide, and here in the U.S. we are paying a terrible price for the lack of managing the Pandemic from the beginning. Outbreaks and deaths continue daily at a record pace with very little relief in sight. Worldwide on November 22, two pharmaceutical companies have applied for emergency approval and an expected third company has shown great results, the actual vaccinations to the general public is far from being a reality. Most optimistic projections would be mid-2021. The production and the logistics of actually getting this to all the population in cities and outstate areas is a task the world has never faced before. The world also has never faced a crisis that is escalating at such an alarming rate and is so dependent upon successful vaccines ASAP.

On March the 20th, 2020, the world was reporting 10,000 deaths. On April 3rd this had risen to 50,000 deaths. 8 days later the death total was 100,000, and by the 25th of April 200,000 had lost their lives. In May/June, no relief was in sight and deaths totaled over ½ million people, from this uncontrolled virus by the end of June. By the end of August, the total had reached 900,000 and by November 1.3 million people had lost their lives. The trends appear out of control, and are projected by 2021 to exceed 2 million people. The U.S. which leads all countries by far has recorded 12,387,456 infected cases, 1,129,312 in the last 7 days. The death rate in the U.S. has reached 281,156, with 10,088 the past seven days. In the U.S. there is major concern on the reluctance of the population to adhere to the restrictions being put in place and the response of the people with the upcoming Holiday celebrations. We cannot treat this Holiday period as past holiday periods, and we need to make sacrifices, to keep any hope of getting this under control, health officials are stating. If people in other countries can find a way to adjust their lifestyle to help themselves, and be concerned about everyone around you, then we as Americans can find a way to help each other.

Some additional good news arrived on November 23rd when Astra Zeneca announced their vaccine had passed the 90% success rate and they were proceeding to seek approval for rollout of their vaccine. The advantage they bring to the process is their Vaccine does not require the low temperature controls of Pfizer or BioNTech, previously seeking emergency approvals. Astra Zeneca has not only proceeded to secure a vaccine awaiting approvals, but has manufacturing capabilities in process which will enable Astra Zeneca to produce millions of available dosages by January 2021.

As the news of the great success of this third vaccine showed promise, the excitement lasted for only a short time as Astra Zeneca admitted it probably made a mistake in the dosage received by some of the study participants. The admission erodes some of the confidence scientists and industry experts had in Astra Zeneca and the release of the data.

Direct Impact on Individuals Going into Holidays

POST THANKSGIVING

While National, and State recommendations to avoid large gatherings, and requests to rethink travel during the Thanksgiving week, once again the self-centered society of the U.S. filled the airports, with over 3 million on airplanes and celebrated like it can't happen to us. The numbers of people Friday through Wednesday totaled 900,000 to 1 million per day. Reports that planes were packed in many cases with center seats occupied and masks ineffective while passengers ate and drank. Without question there will be a price to pay for ignoring procedures, and impacting other members of the society. What we will soon learn is the people who refuse to comply with medical direction and science, will lead this nation into new levels of infections and deaths within the next few weeks, and then probably step it up a notch and repeat the disregard at Christmas. As Thanksgiving Day passed in the U.S. with lower infected rates, the numbers were expected to escalate dramatically over the weekend as testing on Thanksgiving and Friday was basically low as staff had holiday schedules, and testing was reduced. The Pandemic worldwide continued to escalate and expansion of restrictions impacted virtually every country and every citizen.

In Germany, lockdown restrictions were imposed in November on restaurants and bars, as deaths totaled 410 in a 24-hour period, up 249 from the previous day. This daily total was the deadliest day since the beginning of the pandemic and brought the death toll to 14,771. 18,633 new cases were reported in that 24-hour period bringing the total being reported to 961,320.

At the Vatican in Italy as Pope Francis prepares to elevate 13 clerics to the College of Cardinals, the elite group of red-robbed churchmen whose primary task is to elect a new pope. The Santa Marta Hotel was built to sequester cardinals during papal elections, but is now being used to sequester soon to be Cardinals as they await the weekend ceremony to their new appointment in quarantine confined to their quarters with room meal delivery. Two candidates will participate via zoom, as due to travel restrictions, travel was not possible. Italy is in the 2nd major wave and the Vatican is in modified lockdown prior to the celebration. Typically, this was a time of celebration, with huge crowds and parties and gatherings of family members, and parishioners celebrating their Cardinals elevation.

In North Korea, Korean Leader Kim, has ordered two people killed, banned fishing at sea, and locked down the capitol Pyongyang as part of some frantic efforts to slow the Covid virus and its economic impact to the country. One of his lawmaker's, indicated Kim is displaying excessive anger and taking irrational measures over the pandemic and its economic impact.

In the U.S. Los Angeles County, which is the nation's most populous county, announced a new stay at home order, as cases surged out of control, banning most gatherings but stopping short of full shutdowns on retail stores and other non-essential businesses. Their 5-day average of new cases has risen to almost 4,800 cases.

A border closure has been in place between the U.S. and Canada since mid-march and has been extended through at least December 21st, but many feel it could extend well into 2021. Essential workers have been able to cross for employment but other Canadian citizens can only cross with strict restrictions and quarantine periods required. With the rise in infections, neither country is willing to open any possibility of virus expansion which they can't control.

As case rates around the World continue to escalate, the reported cases have many variations due possibly to transparencies and methods of tracking. The U.S., Russia and France report case infection rates are doubling every 2 months, Brazil every 5 months, Canada and Germany every month and China reports a doubling every 14 years. Likewise, while the U.S reports 820 deaths per 1 million people, Brazil 809, Spain 955, France 798, U.K 853, China is reporting 3. Clearly the worldwide community is not getting an accurate reading of the extent of devastation this virus is causing.

It's very easy to see from the worldwide infection summaries and the recorded death totals, the free world as such, appears to be very transparent versus China, and controlled countries of the world. China for example is country of the origination of the disease and has the largest population base in the world, and yet the reported data on the pandemic's impact on their people in infections and deaths, is obviously under reported, to give the world a false sense of their ability to control the virus. Their lack of transparencies on information releases, impacts working with the world community to measure the extent and control of this world-wide disaster. This has been the case with the Chinese Government since the announcement of the outbreak early in 2020. Reports now indicate the virus was well known to the medical community early in December of 2019, but kept internally. A confidential report in early December reflects there were eight Doctors who reported concerns about an illness, but were reprimanded for spreading rumors. One of those Doctors later died from the virus but the Hospital was instructed not to say anything. The origin of the virus remains a mystery as 2020 comes to an end. One of the original theories was that it originated in bats and was transmitted to humans. That has never been confirmed as they have been unable to confirm bats are infected in the Wuhan area. They only sign of any virus contamination was in sewage in the Wuhan area. As this was further being researched, a similar sewage contamination was discovered in Barcelona earlier in 2020 which may indicate the virus did not originate in China but was in other parts of the world near the same time. Also, of interest as worldwide numbers are released is the impact of the pandemic as it effects the individual Worldwide countries population. Taking two countries with similar infection totals, December 1st, Germany with 1,152,283, and Mexico with 1,144,643. The death totals for the two countries are completely different and should be something the WHO may be evaluating very closely. Germany has 18,340 deaths or 21.82 per 1 million population, while Mexico has 108,173 deaths or 85.72 per 1 million people. Many factors could conceivably come into play, of restrictions imposed, living conditions of families, employment protections, available protection equipment, available hospital care, and staff as well as others. Much could also be said of the U.S and the individual States, where infection rates and death totals have no correlation, yet one would look at individual States as having a more closely defined set of numbers. If one would look at two neighboring States, Wisconsin and Michigan, Wisconsin has 426,534 reported case infections and 3,781 reported deaths, while neighboring Michigan has 420,286 case infections but 10,117 reported deaths. Many factors contributed to the variance in the U.S. The political environment caused more disarray than anyone could believe. With no leadership at the Federal level, States either attempted to establish controls with huge opposition from millions who followed the blind direction of our President, or tried to mandate restrictions without total compliance. In short, the leaders of the States were handicapped and implemented controls with limited support.

Three U.S. States by December have infections exceeding 1 million people, and over 20,000 deaths.

December 2020

As December 2020 arrives, the virus remains far from under control worldwide, and while restrictions being implemented virtually everywhere in the world, it seems to be doing little to slow the rate of infections, and the resulting death rates. As the virus enters its 11th month, the number of infections and deaths is staggering, and the daily expansion of infections and deaths, leaves everyone in a critical state of uncertainty, of any future solution and return to a normal life.

DECEMBER 3rd VIRUS INFECTIONS   DEATH TOTALS

TOTAL INFECTIONS	INFECTIONS	TOTAL DEATHS	DEATHS
LAST 24-HOURS		LAST 24-HOURS	
GLOBAL	65,686,172	669,836	1,514,549	11,821
U.S.	14,464,000	238,540	281,798 2,874	2,874

VACCINE PROGRESS DECEMBER 2020

Three Drug-makers are either in final stages. or in final consideration for emergency approval. Giant Pharmaceutical Pfizer and its German partner BioNTech, a Biotechnology firm

Moderna, and the University of Oxford partnered with Astra Zeneca. Both the Pfizer and Moderna are close to Emergency approval by the FDA, and anticipate providing 40 million doses by the end of the year, enough for injecting 20 million people. The virus distribution is fairly well defined after months of discussion. The US has about 200 million people who could be included in a priority status starting with health care workers, first responders, teachers and essential workers. Senior residents in long term, and people with health concerns would receive the first vaccinations. The Pfizer vaccine requires shipment frozen to -70 degrees Celsius and maintained under refrigeration for no more than 5 days, and the second injection three weeks after the first injection. The Moderna vaccine is stored frozen at -20 degrees, and can be kept at refrigerator temperatures for one month. The Astra Zeneca entry can be stored at refrigeration temperature for up to six months, which would make distribution far easier to distribute and administer worldwide.

Pfizer is currently shipping vaccine in Britain to 50 Hospital units and vaccinations are due to begin by December 8th in England, Scotland, Ireland, and Wales, to a defined succession of the population: By December 6th, the progression of the virus in these countries is enormous with 1,723,242 people infected, and 61,245 deaths. In the past 24 hours there was recorded 17,242 new cases, and 231 deaths. 225,504 are currently hospitalized an increase of 1,444 the past 24 hours.

Planned vaccine schedule beginning December 8th

1st Residents of long-term care facilities and care workers

2nd Everyone 80 and over and frontline health care workers and social care workers.

3rd People 75 and over

4th People 70 and over

With the World watching, Britain has dubbed the start of the immunization program as V-Day, a nod to the triumphs of World War II. Around 800,000 doses of the vaccine were expected to be in place to begin the historic beginning of the massive program. Vaccines will be administered at the designated hospitals. Speculation surrounds the Royal family as to whether Queen Elizabeth 94, and Prince Phillip 99, would be vaccinated and made public reassuring the public the vaccine was safe.

While the nursing homes residents were top priority on the independent Joint committee on Vaccinations and immunizations, they will not be getting the vaccines in the first wave. (British version not getting it straight away) The vaccine is packed in 975 doses, and dividing the packs of doses, and shipping to the individual nursing homes, needs an approved method up splitting up the packs for safe storage and controlled delivery.

As the vaccinations began in Britain, the process unfortunately received a temporary setback as two nurses had a reaction to the injection. Immediate action by Pfizer announced it possibly triggered a reaction due to a certain drug being taken by the individuals. The two nurses with the reactions were quickly treated, and have no long term, or serious reactions to the drug. The reactions from these two individuals gives direction to those taking the drug, and the medical community administering the vaccinations. The Medical Regulator from Britain warned that people with serious respiratory reactions, should not take the vaccine from Pfizer and Biotech, until investigators were able to evaluate the cause of the reactions of the two people in question.

While England and the U.K. moved quickly to seek emergency approval and begin actual vaccination on December 7th, their earlier departure from the EU has left the other European countries positioned far behind in the approval process, and the actual vaccine acquisition process. With limited production, and the growing demands of the UK and the US, the EU's drug regulators won't be making any decision until after the first of 2021, which puts actual injections of a vaccine towards the end of January more of a reality. And that's assuming dosages are available for shipment in January. A further delay exists for some EU countries, like, Germany, France and Italy, who will be delayed further, as they require approval individually, by their own agencies prior to actual vaccinations to their population.

Canada has given emergency approval to the Pfizer vaccine, and is expected to receive 249,000 doses before the end of the month, and begin vaccinating the Canadian population. Israel and the UAR announced they will begin vaccinating their residents beginning December 27th.

Both Russia and China have started vaccinations on an emergency approval basis with China having 5 different vaccines from four producers. It involved testing of these vaccines in more than one dozen countries. Russia on Saturday December 5th, began vaccinating thousands of doctors, teachers, and others, at centers in Moscow, with its Sputnik V vaccine. Clearly the scientific community has responded to the Pandemic at an amazing pace, all over the World. For the first time in many years, the world community has a common goal, which could potentially become a unifying common denominator, in developing a peaceful world community.

BARCELONA SPAIN MEDICAL STUDY

More than 1,000 Barcelona residents, gathered on Saturday December 12th to participate in a medical study to evaluate the effectiveness of same day COVID screening to safely hold cultural events.

After passing an antigen screening, 500 of the volunteers, were randomly selected to enjoy a free concert inside Barcelona's Apola Theatre. The other 500 were sent home. They will form a control group that will allow the organizers to analyze if there was any contagion inside the concert hall despite the antigen tests. The antigen tests are not as accurate as other types of testing, but produces results within 15 minutes compared to several hours, or days as required from other testing. The antigen testing, it was felt it could be an effective tool for handling large events safely until widespread vaccines are widespread enough to control the virus. The 500 that were allowed into the concert were required to wear masks other than in a downstairs bar, and participated in a 5-hour concert without social distancing, and mingled on the dance floor similar to a real concert atmosphere.

The 1,000 volunteers will also undergo two PCR tests, which will have a higher capacity to detect the virus than the antigen test. The first on the Saturday before the concert and the second 8 days after the concert. The PCR testing will allow investigators to determine if any infected people got by the antigen testing, and infected people at the concert. Spain remains under limited restrictions for the Pandemic, which has killed 47,600 residents.

The Virus continues to spread at uncontrollable rates world-wide. December 10th recorded a total of 69,354,040 case infections and 1,577,875 deaths. Never in the history of man has this level of devastation existed. The US continues to lead the World in case infections, and death totals. By mid-December the U.S. reported almost 6 million people have been infected with close to 300,000 deaths, and the number of case infections is doubling every two months. The U.S. saw 3,000 deaths in a single day this past week setting a record, and exceeding daily totals from last spring. Daily case infections exceed 200,000 on average. and hospitalizations with 105,00 patients currently admitted, is the highest on record. Los Angeles County, the nations most populated County is showing a devastating increase in deaths, with over 8,000 in a single day.

On December 11th, the U.S. recorded one day deaths of over 3,124. This total surpassed the total number of deaths on the opening day of the Normandy invasion, and the loss of life on 9/11. Also, over 1 million new cases have been recorded in the last five days. Clearly the spread of this disease is totally out of control in the U.S. More than 106,000 Americans are currently hospitalized recuperating from the virus, which in many States and cities has the health communities at a breaking point. Patients diagnosed with the virus in parts of South Dakota and Wyoming are being transferred to Hospitals in Denver Colorado, in some cases 400 miles away. This means an EMS crew and an ambulance are out of the system for over a day, and the families of the patients are left helpless. It has been said that patients have gone from thinking this was a hoax, to "WOW ", this is real. People need to understand that at the end of the day, the virus doesn't care if you believe in it or not.

Hospitals are unable to manage the increasing patient load. More than 1/3 of all Americans, are living in an area where an intensive care bed is unavailable. In New Mexico officials are evaluating the patient load, and with no ICU beds available, are permitting medical personnel to ration care, based on who they expect to survive. In California where a shortage of hospital beds initiated a lockdown in much of the state, over 10,000 COVID patients are now hospitalized. This is 70% higher than the total two weeks ago and the impact of Thanksgiving is still unknown.

Clearly the lack of direction and the attitude of the American public, feeds the virus in the U.S. The virus initially appeared to be one which spared the smaller communities, but is now out of control in smaller communities. As the population deems mask wearing. and imposed regulations contrary to their beliefs, and their individual rights, they share with all others a responsibility to protect others, and be part of the community, rather than be a defiant citizen claiming individual rights. Public officials in many states and communities are threatened, as they attempt to impose mask wearing, initiate safety measures, closures and curfews to protect the citizens. Actual bodily threats, are being made to public officials. Clearly the American public cannot work together to resolve anything that is not deemed well for the individual person. In contrast to the rest of the World we have become a me society. The "me" if left to expand will destroy this democracy. In Boise Idaho, three protesters were arrested outside the home of a County Commissioner on a anti mask protest group rally. She stated, I don't recognize this place anymore. There is an ugliness and cruelty in our national rhetoric that has reached a fevered pitch here at home, that should worry us all. To further complicate the unrest in this country is the refusal by the outgoing President Donald Trump, who refuses to accept the fact he lost the election, and is to leave office on January 20th 2021. He has a staff of lawyers who continue to pursue every ridiculous avenue and means, to try and get a court to agree that he his has some sort of claim of fraud, that cost him the election. While every attempt has failed and he has no valid claim, his non-stop dialog has millions stirred up, and protests will be, and are uncontrollable. The protests gather multitudes of people spreading the virus, rather than working with the community to reduce exposure.

GOOD NEWS

The FDA on December 11th approved the Pfizer vaccine in the U.S, and shipments of the vaccine are to begin on December 12th followed by vaccinations to health care workers, and nursing homes expected as early as Monday December 14th. Initial doses are scarce as several countries are competing to receive what is a rationed supply, until production is able to adequately supply the needs worldwide. The World desperately requires multiple vaccines, to have enough to supply the needs of the world. Pfizer was the first to emerge from that worldwide race based on rigorous scientific testing to record a record setting achievement. Several other vaccines are under testing and could be vaccine options in the very new future.

The U.S, will receive about 3 million doses to be distributed around the country on the initial shipment, with another 3 million held in reserve for the second vaccination. On Monday December 14th, 145 Hospitals and distribution points will receive doses, Tuesday an additional 76 and Wednesday 66 more. The U.S. is also considering a second vaccine by Moderna which is expected to receive approval before the years end. If the Moderna vaccine is approved, and shipments are received, the U.S. is expected to vaccinate 20 million doses in December, another 30 million in January, and 50 million in February 2021. The Johnson and Johnson entry is expected to complete it's testing in January and could be approved for shipment and vaccination early in 2021. The transportation of the vaccine is critical and must meet very strict transportation regulations. UPS and FEDEX have created special transportation equipment to keep the doses at -94 degrees. The Moderna vaccine will also need to be refrigerated, but not to the degree of the Pfizer entry. The Pfizer vaccine needs to be packed in dry ice with a GPS tracker, to monitor temperature and track the shipments. Both of the vaccines will require two individual vaccinations, The Pfizer entry at 21 days, the Moderna entry at 28 days. Because the vaccines are so new, researchers do not know how long the protections will last. The SARS-CoV-2 virus is studded with proteins which it uses to enter human cells. These so-called spike proteins make a tempting target for vaccines, and both of the current vaccines, are built on the genetic instructions of the virus to build these spike proteins.

The U.S. and the World desperately need the virus shipments and the possible relief anticipated if the vaccinations are to begin a change to the current ugly trends. The week ending December 13th marked the worst week since the beginning of the virus with 71,866,583 recorded infections, 517,175 in the last 24 hours. The worldwide death count reached 16,222,485, with 197,362 in the past 24 Hours. In virtually every part of the world, the virus continues totally out of control. The vaccine arrival this week is desperately needed, and could not arrive soon enough. While each of the States have individual vaccine priority regulations, in most cases the health care community, and nursing home residents/workers will receive priority, along with EMT emergency personnel. In Minnesota, the vaccine arrived at the Veterans Hospital in Minneapolis, and distribution to statewide Health facilities began immediately. Vaccinations started immediately upon arrival of the vaccine at prearranged health care sites.

The political environment continues to be a stress for everyone who has responsibility of not only trying to control the progression of the disease, but are walking a fine line to keep people safe, while maintaining the economy. In most states, restrictions have been put in place for non-essential business operations, meaning in most states restaurants and bars are closed to the public, with take out only. The Service community is very upset demanding they be allowed to reopen, and are bringing numerous legal actions to reopen. The Governor in Minnesota has set Wednesday the 16th of December to announce future restriction plans, and groups are forming to reopen on their own, regardless of the restriction plans and face whatever action follows. Clearly everyone sees the situation differently, and don't want to comply until they are facing their own death.

In major cities in the U.S drastic controls have been put in place out of uncontrollable increases in infections and deaths. In New York City all Restaurants and bars are closed, as is Broadway. In L.A similar controls are in place with lockdowns and travel restrictions, throughout the otherwise affluent business community.

While the U.S struggles with the restrictions, countries around the world continue to control expansion of the virus. In England, the capitol of London has announced the highest level of restrictions to begin Wednesday December 16th due to new wave of infections, which in some areas is doubling every seven days. The Health Secretary said swift action is needed as they are assessing a new strain of the virus. They are detecting this strain that has been identified in over 1,000 cases, and the initial analysis is this variant is growing faster than other variants. This new variant has been detected in the South of England, in about 60 different local authority areas. Vaccinations are ongoing in England with the Pfizer vaccine which started December 8th to destined locations. Dosages have also arrived to cover the second injections scheduled in three weeks.

December 15th Worldwide Pandemic Controls

RANDOM SELECTED COUNTRIES

EU Countries. Most EU countries entered lockdowns at some point during November and are now in "lockdown light mode" where some restrictions have been lifted depending on the progression of the infection rate. Many continue to curb the movement of people, while planning to allow celebration of Christmas on a small scale with close family. The EU is using a traffic light map from the European Centre for disease control, as a guideline to limit travel from the countries designated as red. Negative COVID tests are being required from arrivals from those countries.

AUSTRIA- Came out of lockdown on December 7th but its restaurants and hotels will stay closed until January 6th (except for business travelers.) A curfew is in effect between 8 pm and 6am. Medical certificates are required from most countries prior to entering with negative COVID test results, or a ten-day Quarantine must be undertaken.

BELGIUM – Outside travel from non-EU countries is prohibited. All passengers arriving by land or sea, must complete a public health Passenger Locator Forum, and give it to border authorities. Anyone arriving from the red zone of the EU must go into Quarantine for ten days, but can test out in seven days with a negative test. Over Christmas guests can be invited to celebrate in the garden, but only one at a time is allowed to enter the house to use the bathroom.

DENMARK- The shutting of bars and gyms has been extended to 31 additional municipalities. Approximately 79% of the population is now affected by the lockdown which will stay in place until January 3rd, 2021.

FRANCE- Lightened its lockdown in December by allowing shops to reopen, but residents need to complete an attestation form to leave the house for more than 3 Hours. The State curfew will be lifted on December 24th, but not On New Year's Eve. Bars Restaurants and Ski Resorts are shut down until January 20th. Ski Resorts in Switzerland will remain open, which presents a border problem, and will require border stops. An action has been presented in the French courts as Restaurants and Ski Resorts challenge to overturn the Government's decision to keep them closed.

GERMANY- They recorded 180 infections per 100,000 people up from 149 one week ago. Also 952 people had died, far greater than the previous one-day record of 598. They have been in a light lockdown for the past six weeks, where all bar and restaurants have been closed, as have other public spaces. Over Christmas, members of one household will be allowed to meet up with other households to celebrate, but are asked to self-isolate before and after such gatherings. However, the Government is considering putting the country into a hard lockdown which would close shops, schools, and day care centers from December 16th until January. Hotels can only allow people to stay, if they are traveling for essential purposes. Ski resorts are closed until January 10th

GREECE- On December 7th, Greece extended its lockdown until January 7th whereby all schools, restaurants, bars, and courts, will be shut down. A night time curfew will be into effect from 9 pm to 5 am.

ITALY- Christmas markets have been banned, and travel throughout Italy is not currently allowed. The government has asked people not to go skiing, fearing it would spread the virus through the alpine area.

NETHERLANDS–With 24 people being admitted to intensive care every day, the Netherlands has extended its lockdown through the festive period, which means that no more than 3 visitors a day in homes, and restaurants and cafes and bars will remain closed. Everyone is encouraged to work from home and non-essential travel should be avoided.

SPAIN- The State is under a state of emergency putting the entire country under a nationwide curfew from 11pm. to 6am. Between December 23rd and January 6th 2021, gatherings of people is limited to 10 with strict regulations. Ski resorts will be allowed to stay open, but under strict regulations.

SWITZERLAND-Travel is permitted Between Switzerland and its immediate neighbors, Austria, Italy, Germany and France, but other regions have been designated into a high-risk category.

ENGLAND-They came out of lockdown on December 2nd and classified the country into three tiers, each with different restrictions. Tier 1 and 2, have reduced restrictions, tier 3 all entertainment venues are closed down, and hospitality businesses are closed except for takeaway services. On December 18th Prime Minister Boris Johnson created a Tier 4 and announced more aggressive restrictions due to the aggressive rate of infections from a new virus strain in the Southeast of London region, and London proper. The tier 4 places the strictest restrictions regarding travel, and gatherings, impacting Christmas Day. Residents in tier 4 are experiencing this new threat which apparently spreads very rapidly, and scientists have not determined its origin, or how it differs from the current virus. This new restrictive tier will force millions to alter their Christmas plans.

The WHO has been involved in the development of this new strain and is actively working with the scientific community to evaluate the progress, and its impact relative to transmission and the vaccine impact versus other strains.

CHINA – As the world continues to struggle with the rapid increase of infections and deaths, China mysteriously reports minimal, cases of new infections and deaths. With 1,439,323,776 people in the country, and the country where the virus reportedly originated, the number of new cases reported was 23 the past 24 hours for a total of 86,829, and 4,634 total deaths. New cases being reported for a 24-hour period on December 20th worldwide was 295,887, of which China was reporting 23.

Reports have surfaced relative to China's attempt to censor the information regarding this virus since early December 2019. A Chinese doctor in December reported this virus outbreak, but he was silenced and threatened by the police, and accused of peddling rumors. He died and news began to spread of his death possibly from the virus he was communicating. Quickly the Chinese censors began to suppress the information being circulated, and the reporting of his death, they removed his name from any and all social media.

Curbs on media coming out of China began in early January as the virus obviously was beginning to gain legs, but information controls were in place weeks before the outbreak in Wuhan eliminating any chance to warn the World and the WHO. Documents now reveal the Chinese Government in early January 2020 allowed only Government sources to report any activity on the virus, and to play up their ability to control the extent of the virus. Online reports were to play up the heroic efforts of the medical community, as well as the heroic contributions of the communist party. Headlines were to stay clear of the words fatal, or incurable. In hindsight, the world community should have listened more closely to the people from other countries, who exited Wuhan at the outbreak and ultimately were the element to spread worldwide the virus. The controls put in place by the Government were effective, as by the end of February 2020, the death of Dr, Li Wenliang was a forgotten news issue. Based on data being reported and the numbers being shared, the Pandemic impact on the World is far greater than being reported. Of real danger to the world is the new strain discovered in Southeast London that could already be in China and suppression by the Government can't be of assistance to the scientific community and WHO as they attempt to evaluate this new strain of COVID.

USA- Record infections and deaths virtually every day. Over 16.5 million people infected, with over 300,000 deaths. While controls vary by state, restaurants and bars are closed in the majority of the states and gathering restrictions continue to be emphasized, but as with other requests, a large number of people do not follow, and put others at risk. The Thanksgiving fallout has begun, and will again be tested as Christmas and New Year's approach. The good news is vaccinations have begun with the Pfizer entry beginning to be injected, and the Moderna close to approval.

The process of vaccinating in the U.S. beginning December 13th, will focus on health care workers and in many states, move to the thousands of nursing homes and assisted living facilities who have suffered massive infections and deaths nationwide. At least 106,000 residents and staff of long-term care facilities have died from the virus accounting for 38% of the fatalities to date. But as plans are being developed, experts are factoring in what could be a high level of resistance to being vaccinated, starting with the nursing home staff.

The Government has contracted with Walgreens and CVS, to travel to the 75,000 long term care facilities to vaccinate both the staff and the residents. 40,000 of the facilities have opted to work with CVS, and 35,000 with Walgreens. It is up to each state to decide which of the two vaccines to use at the outlets.

In that both require two injections, a return trip will be necessary at each outlet. These two companies have been preparing staff for this assignment and appear to be in position to begin by December 21st, assuming approvals are complete.

The Staff injections can be given in a common area, but the residents will receive theirs in their rooms. The facilities typically have more than one shift of workers on duty so coordination will be needed to insure everyone is covered. The management of the homes face internal difficulty, as if there are any reactions from staff to the injections, it will result in time away from the facility while the employees are recuperating, and they are already experiencing shortage of staff. Many staff have reportedly indicated they will refuse the injections, which creates other issues, as the schedule for the Walgreen/CVS does not have the flexibility to keep returning, especially when the homes are in isolated communities.

The residents present obstacles as well, as when approval is required, a number of the residents lack understanding and or are dealing with memory issues, and approval is required by secondary family members. The logistics of coordinating all of these issues will be a real challenge for nursing care management and facility ownership. As one management person described it, if 10% of the workers call in sick one day, and the residents have resulting issues and are irritated, upset, or are having adverse reactions, you have created the perfect storm.

Many states in the U.S, had established regu-lations which were to either end, or be revised mid- December. In states like Minnesota which had closures for indoor dining and bar closures, there had been major resistance, and operators who chose to defy the mandates and challenge the right of Government to impose these closures. Some in defiance opened and faced penalties. On December 17th the Governor made a minor adjustment to restrictions, but announced restaurants and bars were to remain closed, offering only take out.

The Pandemic remains out of control. The U.S. recorded over 3,000 deaths on December 15th for the third time in less than a week, and infection rates are exceeding to over 220,000 per day. The number of people in the U.S. hospitalized with the virus hit a new high of 113,000. Many areas of the U.S are suffering beyond belief. In California 5,000 body bags are on order and refrigerated trucks are standing by, as the death rate is averaging 163 per day, up from 63 just two weeks ago. Daily case infections have risen to 33,000 per day, up from 14,000 at the beginning of the month. Hospitals are under siege and no end is in sight at this point. Clearly people need to take this more seriously, to ensure controls are in place to capitalize on the vaccine rollout, and to pave the way for its success.

While not receiving a lot of publicity as the virus enters its 10th month, is the fact that over 275,000 prisoners currently are infected with the virus, and over 1,700 have died, and there is no sign of slowing is in sight. New infections hit an all-time high this week. One in every 5 prisoners in State and Federal prisons is testing positive at a rate 4 times the general population. In Kansas, which has the highest rate of infections, over ½ of the prison population is infected. In Arkansas 4 out of every seven have tested positive, and over 50 have died. In many states, on an attempt to reduce exposure, prisoners are released early to avoid crowded conditions. Currently many prisons cannot keep safe conditions due to crowded cafeterias, open cell closures, dorm sleeping accommodations and, in many places, less than perfect health systems, and air filtration. Racial disparities in the criminal justice system, also contribute to the toll the pandemic has taken on the communities of color. Black Americans are incarcerated at 5 times the rates of whites. They are also disproportionately more likely to be infected and hospitalized. The pandemic increases the risk of those who are already at risk. Nationwide, the mortality rate among prisoners is 45 % higher than the general population.

As States begin to vaccinate the residents of their individual states and develop phases for injections, there is a great deal of skepticism as to where residents of a penitentiary, are to be included, to appease the total community

As December moves toward Christmas, the monthly death count has already exceeded the total deaths of November in many states. The total death count in the U.S. week ending December 20th was 323,745 an increase of 341, the past 24 Hrs. Over 18,000,000 have been infected, close to 25% of the world's total.

On December 20th, as countries begin to deal with the possibility of a new virus strain, which apparently is surfacing in London, and the impact of the upcoming Christmas Holiday, the EU nations are beginning to bar travel to the UK. France, Germany, Italy, the Netherlands, Belgium, Austria, Ireland and Bulgaria, have all announced restrictions on UK travel. A total of 40 countries have travel bans in place, as the UK infections are rising at an alarming rate. On one recent day mid-December, they had record infections of 36,800 people. They now have recorded 68,000 deaths, second only to Italy with 69,800.

Studies are underway to better understand how the new virus strain which is sweeping through the south of London, spread so fast, and whether it's related to the variant itself, or a combination of other factors. Currently the new strain appears to be 70% more transmissible than the original COVID-19.

Studies indicate the strain has also been identified in Denmark, the Netherlands and Australia. Virtually every country is carefully watching the progression of the 2nd strain and be ahead of its progress. It's believed the current vaccine will be effective on either of the two current strains. Pandemics in the past have had similar experiences, with new variations surfacing as the virus progresses.

France has banned all travel from the UK, including trucks carrying freight through the tunnel under the English Channel, or from the port of Dover on the south coast. French officials are facing a serious dilemma dealing with the thousands of trucks who used the tunnel on a daily basis. In Germany all flights coming from Britain except cargo flights, were no longer allowed to land. Belgium also issued a flight ban. Air Travel from Netherlands, Ireland, Italy, Israel, South Africa have also added restrictions, and flights from Canada were banned with the exception of cargo planes.

After 3 days of banned travel which impacted truckers who were crossing the English-channel near dover between France and England, restrictions were being revised to allow the trucks to leave England to return to their origination. About 6,000 trucks were denied passage to return to their home countries, which eliminated their chance to spend Christmas with their family. Immediate plans were being initiated to set up COVID testing of the drivers before leaving England, due to the possibility of spreading the new virus, as these drivers returned to their home countries.

England has the majority of its food products brought in from France, Spain, and other EU countries, and faced major shortages in stores, and would soon face an unmanageable dilemma for families. On Christmas eve, trucks began boarding ferries to cross the English Channel, for the first time in four days. About 4,000 of the 6,000 trucks waiting to cross, and their drivers, were parked in an airport area, with little food or accommodations available, and forced to sleep in their trucks for days. It is estimated it will take several more days to clear the logjam, meaning all will miss family Christmas.

Several days earlier, sea, rail, and air routes had opened, but the backlog only began to loosen as authorities developed COVID screening tests. The Government dispatched the military to assist in the testing of travelers.

Other countries mandated testing, to control the possible influx of the new virus. The U.S. began to require all airline passengers arriving from Britain to test negative for the virus within 72 hours of their departure. At least 50 countries have sealed their borders to travel from Britain or imposed restrictions on their arrivals.

In Switzerland authorities are trying to locate 10,000 people who flew in from the UK, since December 14th and is ordering them to quarantine for 10 days. Switzerland is one of the only countries who left their ski resorts open, so they are popular with the other UK countries which had closed their resorts. The quarantine will be closely monitored and violations face a fine of 10,000 francs ($11,275)

Currently the Pfizer vaccine is being widely used across the U.S. and other countries. The 2nd vaccine from Moderna has received emergency approval, and is arriving to be included across the U.S. in vaccinations. The U.S. has reached an additional agreement with Pfizer to ship an additional 100 million doses hopefully to arrive by July 2021. As the vaccination process gains momentum, the hesitancy to receive the vaccine appears to declining. Initially the pronounced resistance to the vaccinations came from the rural residents aged between 30 and 49 who tend to be conservative, and not prone to wearing masks and following directives from Government officials. Also, the black families continue to be the most resistant to being vaccinated, even though they tend to be in the high-risk category. The concern is how it is being distributed, and the equality of the process. The trend seems to be changing and more are becoming responsive to being part of the vaccinated.

As countries around the world begin major vaccination programs, the 2nd world countries are far behind due to their inability to finance the needed vaccines, as they compete with the affluent countries of the world. The ability to compete financially, is not the only problem being faced, it's the logistics involved in distribution, storage, and medical staff to manage the vaccinations. Clearly the world community, and the WHO, need to step up and partner with these countries. If we are to be able successfully to control this pandemic, we are dependent upon a worldwide effort, shared by all countries.

By Christmas day 2020, the impact of the virus on the U.S. population is staggering. A total of 331,116 Americans died from the virus, out of a U.S. population of 330,753,142.

When we consider that the first death from the virus was recorded in Washington State on February 29th; this is a progression of U.S. deaths since that first death.

Total deaths in the U.S. by March 24th 1,000

Total deaths by April 4th 10,000

Total deaths by April 23rd 50,000

Total deaths May 23rd 100,000

Total deaths September 21st 200,000

Total deaths December 14th 300,000

11 days later on December 26th 331,116 deaths have died from the virus.

Meanwhile by December 26th, 9,547,9255 vaccine doses have been distributed in the U.S. and 1,944,585 first doses had been administered by December 26th.

As much of the country continues to experience spiking infection rates, the upper Midwest who had been experiencing a devastating surge of the virus has been given some cautious relief. Health officials however worry that the Christmas holiday travel, could reignite the worst outbreaks of the season. The weeks before the Thanksgiving holiday recorded the highest infection rates in the country, in the Midwest, and plains states, stretching hospitals beyond capacity. Since the middle of November, these states have returned to the levels of mid-October. The Governors of the states have been emphatic for the residents to maintain the restrictions in place, and to eliminate holiday travel and gatherings to avoid a renewed outbreak, which would stretch the medical community beyond its capabilities.

The end of year travel however was higher than expected, and poses a significant risk as we head into 2021. Air travel was less than last year, and the risk of traveling by air is low due the controls while in the air, and the air exchange systems on the planes. It's what transpires after the people are off the planes in gatherings, and inside activities, that will create the additional infection spikes. The number of people traveling by car to other states, was estimated at 81 million. While less than last year, health experts are concerned that we are far from being out of the woods with the virus, and having any degree of letdown could be critical.

As the U.S. desperately attempts to secure additional dosages from the two approved vaccines, other manufacturers continue to test, in hopes of rolling out another vaccine to fill the pipeline and reduce the waiting period for the population at large. Currently the Pfizer and the Moderna vaccines are being administered in the U.S. and the UK while Russia has a Sputnik vaccine being widely distributed in Russia and Argentina. China has produced a vaccine and is proceeding to vaccinate the Chinese people on a rapid schedule. They have an additional three vaccines in tests in other countries. The EU had, as a group, agreed to begin vaccinations in 2021, with a unified plan, but Germany, Hungary, and Slovakia, began injections as soon as the vaccines arrived, upsetting the rollout plans of the EU nations. The comment from the German health director was, "every day we wait is one day too many".

The desperate need to vaccinate the entire world, puts extreme pressure on the supply train and the demands that additional vaccines be available and in the system. Currently the two approved vaccines available in the U.S., Pfizer and Moderna, are Genetic code vaccines which means a genetic code is injected to coat the coronavirus, a messenger RNA, to induce the body to produce some harmless spike protein, to prime the immune system to react if it comes in contact with the real virus. Both of these vaccines must be kept frozen, which makes the distribution in many parts of the world difficult, and in some cases impossible. Astra Zeneca has a vaccine in final testing and on schedule for approval in the U.S. Another vaccine has tests underway in Europe from a German company, Cure-Vac and has possibilities. Novavax is pursuing other technology which needs normal refrigeration, and is in late-stage study in Britain and South Africa. It currently is recruiting additional volunteers in the U.S. and Mexico. Another entry gaining legs is the Johnson and Johnson entry, which requires only one dosage. Hopefully one or more of these entries receives the required approvals and contributes to the needed vaccine requirements.

As 2021 is a few days away, the new strain of virus first detected in the London area, continues to spread at an alarming rate and has about ½ of England in strict lockdown. People have been ordered to stay at home, but the rate of infections continues to skyrocket and spreading now throughout England. Hospitals are treating more patients than at any time during the Pandemic. The number of new infections daily sets new records. Scientists have determined the new virus strain, apparently is driving the new rate of infections. Over 53,000 cases were reported in a single day on December 29th, the highest one-day total in Britain to date. Over 20,000 are hospitalized and being treated for COVID.

While England attempts to control the spread of this new strain from within, other countries are initiating measures to reduce the influx into their countries by barring flights from the UK. It is not uncommon for a virus to change as it moves through a populated base, as it reproduces itself. Actually, new variants have been detected in China since the virus was first detected almost 1 year ago. If the virus were to have significant mutation changes, it could begin to impact the success of the vaccine created for control. At this point Scientists do not see this as an issue with the current virus. However there exists the possibility other variants can surface and may respond differently.

The current new variant detected in the UK known as B.1.1.7, has also been found in Canada, Italy, India, and the United Arab Emirates. On December 29th, the first case was confirmed in the U.S. where in Colorado, a man was diagnosed with the new strain, but had no travel history to the UK. Another man from another county also was being diagnosed, who happened to work in the same county as the confirmed case. On December 31st, an infection believed to be of the variant was reported in California, indicating the new strain may be working its way through the U.S. Scientists are working to determine tracking of these two individuals in Colorado, to determine a possible infection trail. Another strain of variant has been detected in South Africa, known as 501.V2, and is believed to be the cause of recent infection spikes, hospitalizations, and deaths in South Africa. Clearly the road ahead for the health scientists is not a smooth transition.

As England attempts to control the spread of the new variant virus identified south of London, Britain became the first country to authorize AstraZeneca's vaccine on December 30th as a weapon to use against the out-of-control virus sweeping the country. The plan now in England is to vaccinate as many as possible, using both the Pfizer and the Astra Zeneca.

The Astra Zeneca entry is a welcome addition, due its low cost and the ease of handling the vaccine. The second shot can be given four to 12 weeks giving more time than the current vaccines to complete the vaccination cycle.

This action by Britain could potentially motivate the WHO to give approval to this virus entry, which would clear the vaccine for use in a global effort to help poor countries. The low cost, the refrigeration requirements, and ease of distribution offers the underdeveloped countries a path out of the pandemic. Astra Zeneca plans to manufacture about 3 billion doses by the end of 2021.

China has announced plans to begin expansion globally of a new vaccine produced by Sinopharm, a Chinese controlled firm which had an approval rating of 79%. Plans are to vaccinate 50 million people by the middle of February 2021. The worldwide community is hesitant, due to lack of supporting evidence available. Since the beginning of the Pandemic, China has lacked the compassion to be upfront with the worldwide community, which has resulted in millions of deaths needlessly. In early December 2019, the top Chinese Scientist who was responsible for uncovering the SARS virus, was dispatched to Wuhan in response to a new outbreak of a rare respiratory disease hospitalizing people in Wuhan. After returning to Beijing to sound the alarm, no communication was announced to the worldwide community, for 25 days which meant it was mid-January before the WHO could begin any involvement in developing plans to spread the alarm and begin plans to develop corrective action. Even as 2020 comes to an end, China has been less than transparent about the extent of the virus in China, and the success of vaccination progress. As worldwide numbers are communicated on a daily basis to the WHO, the numbers are understated, as countries like China and also Russia are less than open about extent of the virus and control progress. Russia within the past week announced the infection rates and death rates, had been underreported and were at least 30 % higher than they previously reported.

2020 ends, with the deadliest monthly period on record worldwide. Hope is on the horizon the vaccine expansion and new vaccine entries will begin to control this deadly disease. Complete control will depend on a cooperative effort of the worldwide community, and universal acceptance of vaccinations by the residents of all countries in our world.

2021

As 2021 begins, 2020 ended with the deadliest, most infectious month in history. In the U.S. 6.4 million new cases were confirmed in the month of December, resulting in over 20 million people infected since the first case was reported in early 2020. 77,000 deaths were confirmed in December, bringing the death rate to over 346,000 people in the U.S. ending 2020. 1 out of 17 Americans have tested positive with the COVIC virus.

Areas of the U.S. which at some point, appeared to have controls in place to maintain the spread, have now become areas with the virus out of control. California, the most populous state in the U.S. has infection rates out of control, with hospitals struggling to manage the influx of not only COVIC patients, but the general needs of emergency care, and general hospitalizations. Hospitals have moved patients to hallways, gift shops, cafeterias, meeting rooms, and in many cases left patients in the ambulance for care as there was no place else available at the Hospital. Records are being set daily for case infections, with January 1st recording 585 deaths in a single day. California joined New York and Texas, in reaching over 25,000 deaths from COVID. Experts contend several factors have contributed to the unmanageable spike in the progression of the virus. Thanksgiving holiday travel, social gatherings, and fatigue from people who cannot see beyond the current isolation restrictions.

Also, the detection of the new variant in Southern California could be contributing, although it's not clear at this point how widespread that may be. Based on the recent activity, another massive surge is possible after the fallout from Christmas and New Year activity.

Worldwide, the pandemic spared no populated region of the world, with 218 countries, reporting infections and deaths from COVID-19. The WHO is reporting 81,947,503 confirmed infections through December 2020, with 1,833,583 confirmed deaths. As the New Year begins, several additional countries are now reporting case infections from the new variant of the original COVID virus, which was first recorded in London, and quickly had spread through England. New Year's Eve celebrations in France, and Belgium, as well as a Trump black tie event in Florida which ignored restrictions, and went on without masks and distancing. It is estimated we will have a resulting spike in infections due to people ignoring restrictions that were in place for not only their own good, but for the health of others.

Based on the first few days of 2021, the virus is progressing at record levels, while countries around the world attempt to expand vaccinations, and control not only the original virus but the expansion of the new virus variants. In the U.S., an infection in New York, indicates the new variant previously detected in Colorado, Florida and California, has now spread to additional areas of the U.S. All mutants appear to be the version that has been circulating in England.

Britain meanwhile became the first country to begin vaccinations with the new Astra Zeneca vaccine, ramping up its campaign which began December 8th with the Pfizer vaccine. England is experiencing soaring infection rates, brought in part by the new variant discovered in southern London. More than 1 million people have now been infected in England with Prime Minister Boris Johnson declaring a national lockdown until at least mid–February. Britain is now recording over 50,000 new cases per day, for the last six days, meaning at least 1 person out of every 50 in England now has COVID-19, and deaths have surpassed 75,000, one of the highest in Europe.

Elsewhere in Europe as 2021 begins, France is under fire for slow rollouts and delays. Initially France took a very cautious approach recording only 500 vaccinated the first week. The slow rollout has been blamed on mismanagement, staffing shortages, holidays, and a complex compliance procedure, described as more complex than buying a car. Frances 500 vaccinations compares to over 200,000 in Germany and 100,000 in Italy. India has approved the Astra Zeneca vaccine and will begin an aggressive program to vaccinate it's 1.9 billion people.

By January 10th 2021, barely 1 year after COVID-19 surfaced in China, the pandemic has accelerated to more than 1.9 million deaths, and nearly 90 million case infections despite restrictions and lockdowns and the development of vaccines. In the past three months, the death toll has nearly doubled and total cases have jumped 2 ½ times. The doubling and acceleration totals become more concerning when you view the actual numbers, October 10th 2020 deaths totaled 1,079,984, three months later the total was 1,939,040. Cases recorded were 38,158,808 on October 10th 2020, and 3 months later total 90,363,015. Both are staggering and devastating progressions.

While the case and the death rates mount, the progress of vaccines and actual vaccinations worldwide are showing signs of promise. In addition to the Pfizer, and Moderna approvals, Astra Zeneca is being shipped to many countries and the Johnson and Johnson entry is in final stages for approval. As the vaccinations continue to expand to the 3rd world countries, the worldwide effort seems to be on track. While the progress of the vaccines is a positive sign, the new variant which started in London has now reached several countries, and has been recorded in eight U.S. states by January 10th. Reports the current vaccine will be as effective as the original strain gives hope, we are not in a start over mode.

WORLDWIDE CASES AND DEATHS January 10, 2021

AREA	CASES REPORTED	TOTAL DEATHS
Globally	90,363,015	1,939,040
U.S.	22,451,123	376,521
INDIA	10,466,545	151,184
BRAZIL	8,079,450	202,176
RUSSIA	3,401,954	61,837
UK	3,072,349	81,431
FRANCE	2,767,312	67,599
TURKEY	2,326,256	22,807
ITALY	2,257,866	78,394
SPAIN	2,050,360	51,834
GERMANY	1,914,328	41,061

In Sweden which had resisted lockdowns and legislative efforts to require face masks, has now given parliament the authority to impose regulations to stem the spread of the disease. An emergency law was passed to allow the Government to limit the number of people in stores, and impose regulations with the ability to fine those not complying. The country has 93 deaths per 100,000 people, less than Britain with 120 per 100,000 but more than its neighbor Norway.

In the U.S., originally New York was an uncontrolled state which eventually was brought to manageable levels, and now California has a sustained surge which has put the state in crisis, which is overwhelming intensive care facilities, emergency ambulance services, funeral homes, and hospitals. Emergency rooms have had to shut their doors to arriving ambulances for hours at a time, and needed supplies are at dangerously low levels in the medical wards.

Los Angeles County is reporting a COVID death every eight minutes. It took California 10 months to record 400,000 cases, but one month to add another 400,000 cases. Based on the current trends, 1 in 10 residents will test positive for the virus. Part of the reason for the surge, appears to be the Thanksgiving effect and lack of managing gatherings despite warnings. People just will not comply with the requests by the medical community to help curb the spread.

Of interest is some data on the progression of the disease by ethnic groups, age groups and gender.

CALIFORNIA COVID BREAKDOWN STATISTICS

ETHNICITY	POSITIVE CASES %	DEATHS %
ASIAN	6.4	11.6
BLACK	4.0	6.7
LATINO	55.0	46.7
WHITE	20.0	31.7
MULTI/RACE	1.3	1.1
OTHER	13.3	2.2

GENDER BREAKDOWN CASES	50.8 % Female	47.7 % Male
DEATHS	42.4 %	57.2 %

AGE BREAK-DOWN	CALIFORNIA COVID CASES	DEATHS
0–17	12.3 %	0.0 %
18–49	58.3 %	6.8 %
50–64	19.0 %	18.5 %
65+	10.4 %	74.6 %

In the U.S, 9 days after the ball dropped in Times square in 2021 to welcome in the New Year, more than two million people have tested positive for COVID and more than 24,500 people have died from COVID. Initially it took 90 days to hit 2 million cases, even as the virus was sweeping through nursing homes and swiftly spreading across the country.

While California and the U.S has had an out-of-control progression of the COVID virus, worldwide Ireland is recording the highest increased infection rates in the world. After being viewed as a model of control early in the pandemic, while neighboring countries were only willing to pursue regional restrictions in hotspot areas. Ireland in October, became the first E.U. country to impose a national lockdown, and maintained one of the lowest rates in Europe. In early December the average daily rate of infections was 127 for a 7-day average. In early December they began to lift restrictions reopening restaurants and retail stores, which led to socializing and holiday get togethers. Going into Christmas, they were reporting 10 new virus cases per day per 100,000 residents. This compares to about 66 per 100,000 in the U.S. But 3 weeks later Ireland is reporting more than 132 new cases per 100,000 compared to the less dramatic increase in the U.S, of 75 cases per 100,000. Relaxing the restrictions prior to the Christmas holidays, and the arrival of the new variant created the perfect storm in Ireland. The new variant has exploded in testing, and the latest testing showed 42 out of 92 samples in a recent testing procedure were positive for the new variant. Ireland has a lower intensive care bed capability than most E.U. countries so it imposes an increased risk on their Health care system.

Public Health officials indicate five factors have contributed to the spike in Ireland.

Opening up hospitality in December

Mixing households

People beginning to travel

Noncompliance at funerals and wakes

Entrance of the new variant

You don't go from 400 cases per day to 7,000 per day because of one thing, it takes several things and eliminating one thing probably has little if any impact.

January 2021 Variants of Covid19

According to the WHO in early January there are other types of COVID – 19 variants causing the disease and circulating the globe.

COVID-19 the original variant of the SARS-2 virus that originated in Wuhan China, that began emergence in early January/February 2020.

Cluster 5, A second variant discovered in Denmark in August and September 2020, discovered in mink farms, but had a reduced virus neutralization in humans. To date few cases have been identified and does not appear to spread as widely as its counterparts.

VOC202012/01 UK Variant

Discovered in Southeast England and possessed increased transmissibility than other mutations, but did not appear to increase the severity of the disease. It rapidly spread and is now reported in 31 other countries.

501Y.V2 Variant found in South Africa.

Discovered in South Africa on December 18ᵗʰ 2020, and is rapidly replacing the COVID -19, in African communities.

Japan also has advised the WHO of a new variant detected in four travelers from Brazil in January 2020, which has similarities to the virus variants in Africa and the UK. Japan and the WHO are working to further analyze this variant and the ability of current vaccines to effectively control it.

The U.S. completely lacks any sense of urgency, with the pandemic. The political battle in the U.S. has gone beyond any sense of reasoning. On January 6ᵗʰ, the current President led a mob, unmasked, of his misdirected supporters to storm the U.S. capitol where the members of the house of Representatives were in the process of certifying Joe Biden as the President. Instead of managing the largest issue ever facing this country, the pandemic, the current President leads a group to break into the Nation's Capital, drives the legislatures into hiding in the basement, while the mob breaks into offices and as a result 5 people died. The Nation remains on high alert as within the next week is the inauguration of the new President, and possible massive violence, as the nation tries to proceed with historic events. The only credence to detailing this in a pandemic history, is the Virus is running ramped, while our government is bogged down on a senseless battle to overturn the election. The incoming President has committed to make the pandemic a national priority day 1 of his Presidency, and has people and programs in place to make this his top priority, but the outgoing administration has not been cooperative in sharing government plans.

Since the Thanksgiving and Christmas holiday celebrations, the U.S is paying a terrible price for increased socializing, and a relaxed attitude towards staying safe. On January 14th, the U.S. reported 4,327 deaths in a 24-hr. period, bringing the average for the last 7 days to over 3,300 per day. This compares to just under 700 per day less than 4 months ago. With less than ½ of the month of January passed, January is expected to be the deadliest month of the COVID pandemic. Three states have now exceeded over 30,000 deaths, since the beginning in mid- February 2020. Texas has recorded 30,000 deaths. California exceeds 31,000 deaths and New York has over 40,000 by mid-January.

Meanwhile the United Kingdom is also setting daily death and case infection records, with 1,564 deaths in a 24-hr period on January 13th. A total of 101,160 people has lost their lives in the UK. The UK is now reporting the highest death rate in the world per 1 million people. Hospitals are admitting one person every 30 seconds with the COVID virus, straining equipment, staff, and facilities beyond belief. Since Christmas Day, 15,000 people have sought admission with COVID infections in England. To put it in perspective, that's the equivalent of filling 30 hospitals with COVID patients. Britain is in its 3rd lockdown which is expected to be reviewed in mid-February, at which time Health care workers, venerable workers, and those over 70 should have at least one dosage of vaccine. Britain has approved three vaccines, and is currently vaccinating the Astra Zeneca, the Pfizer, and will add the Moderna in the spring. The goal in Britain is now to have all adults vaccinated by September 1st 2021, with at least one dosage of a vaccine.

By mid-January, over 95,000,000 cases have been confirmed worldwide, with now over 2,000,000 deaths. Of the 95 million cases, over 25 million remain currently infected, and 115,000 are in serious or critical condition. The U.S., Brazil and the UK, continue to be recording the highest case, and death rates, setting new records almost daily. The U.S. by far is posting the largest case and death numbers, virtually setting records daily. Over 205,000 new cases were reported on January 15, and 3,500 deaths in a 24 Hr. period. In most countries, January could be the deadliest month since the beginning of the pandemic.

New Variants of the virus are being discovered in most parts of the world. Some appear to be of the same mutation of the variant found in the UK, but others are emerging based on the rising numbers of infections. With the high rates of infections currently unchecked, it gives the virus ample opportunities to for it to mutate. Medical experts have indicated the only way to stop the spread of new variants, is to stop the spread of the virus. When a coronavirus infects an individual, it enters the cells and makes copies of itself. And every time it copies itself, there's a chance to introduce errors, and as it is replicating in people, it will slowly accumulate mutations. Most times, these mutations or errors, are meaningless, but in some cases, they can give the virus a survival advantage, and make it more contagious. The opposite can also be said, that it can make the virus weaker. Clearly, we are dealing with new strains of the original COVID variant and will undoubtably be encountering more before this is safely under control. In the U.S, Medical professionals are projecting the new variant now identified in many U.S. states, could become the dominant source of infections in the U.S. by March of 2021, and lead to a wrenching surge in cases, further burdening the already overwhelmed hospital and medical facilities. This variant does not appear to be more deadly, but spreads faster and further. Americans need to redouble their efforts with masks, and the other requested protective measures. The action being taken by the Federal Government of surveillance of the spread of the variant, is too little too late. We had advanced warning of this spread from data in the UK, and had an opportunity to be out front of this possible virus activity. But much like the February 2020 response as this was spiraling in China, the administration in 2021, was focusing on trying to create hysteria over the election. The administration beginning 2021 had made claims about the impact of the WARP program, where the president had funded pharmaceutical companies for research, in return for early availability and supply of vaccines. Mid-January, the Federal Government has a confused program of distribution of vaccines to the states, and are leaving the Governors of the states without direction to manage the individual States vaccination needs, and agreed to supplies. Vaccinations are far behind the projections, and progress being accomplished in other countries. The incoming President being inaugurated on Wednesday, has set a goal of 100 million in the first 100 days. Hopefully a more serious management system will be in place beginning with the new administration to implement this goal and begin to take this seriously.

As the new administration prepares to take control of the process, deaths are exceeding 400,000, as the warnings of an expanded highly contagious variant is taking hold. The CDC has warned that the new Variant will probably become the dominant version in the country beginning in March. The CDC said the new variant is about 50% more contagious than the current virus in the U.S. While the new virus does not cause more severe illness, it does cause more hospitalizations, and deaths, simply because it spreads more easily. The U.S. is under tremendous strain with the virus, as the average daily death rate is rising in 30 of the U.S. states.

January 21ˢᵗ 1 Year of Pandemic

January 21ˢᵗ. one year ago, the first case of the COVID-19 virus was confirmed in the U.S, in Seattle, and the nations failure to address the impact of the pandemic started coming into full view. 415,300 people have lost their lives, since 1/21/20, and the death count continues at a record pace, filling hospitals beyond their capacity. The severity of the outbreak can be traced to the political management of the pandemic in the spring of 2020. Health and scientific recommendations were cast aside by the President and his support staff. The individual State Governors of the Political Party in office, blindly attempted to support the Presidents political directions, and ignored the scientific and the medical community. It quickly expanded out of control, and any attempt to rein it back in, was and is, far out of their reach. A couple of days after the inauguration of President Biden and removal of Trump, Dr. Deborah Brix who served as Trumps administrative coronavirus response coordinator, held a news conference to detail the misinformation from the Trump administration. From the outset she contends the progress against the pandemic, was impeded by the inconsistent and inept public messaging that played down the gravity of the pandemic, and the need for safety precautions.

The message being communicated in the White House was, it was a hoax. Any efforts by her or Dr. Fauci to detail scientific evidence was omitted in the White House communications, to the point neither had any input, and in fact were being censored by the White House. She indicated she then began road trips to meet with various State Governors, so in being out of the White House, it gave her freedom from administration censorship. Both she and Dr Fauci were no longer included in White House briefings. She indicated Vice President Pence was aware of her actions. She was criticized for misleading the information going to the White House, but contends she had no idea where the charts were coming from. She became viewed as part of the Trump apparatus, and was often ignored if she attempted to communicate information deemed in conflict to Trumps internal group. She and one of her staff were the only ones who regularly wore masks and attempted to take safety precautions on a regular basis.

CHINA YEAR 2

More than 1 year ago the world watched with uncertainty, as the Government in China announced the outbreak of a new sirs type virus that was ravaging in Wuhan China. It was highly infective and out of control. By the time the WHO had any chance to act, the Government of China had closed entrance to and out of Wuhan. The mass of people leaving Wuhan when the virus was spreading took with them the virus, which ultimately infected the entire world. While the world was united in an attempt to control this virus, China was determined to control their ownership of the virus and ignored world attempts to share data and find means of control. As countries around the world were in disbelief of the volumes of their new infections and daily total deaths, China continued to report miniscule numbers, indicating they were well ahead of the curve in controlling the virus, and were not recording huge increases of new infections and deaths. Consider the January 21st data in which the countries of the world, record major new infections and new deaths. Data from China, reflects the apparent data inaccuracies. A comparison of data from the U.S and China reported January 21st 2021

U.S. reported cases, a total of 24,998,975, 168,930 on the most recent day. 415,894 reported deaths, 3,785 on the most recent day.

China 88,701 Reported cases, 4,635 deaths, daily data is not reported.

Based on the non-reporting of the country where the virus started, it would indicate the worldwide totals are far underestimated, and the pandemic is beyond our expectations.

U.S. HOSPITALIZATION CRISIS MID JANUARY

One year after the first infection in the U.S, 130,000 people were in Hospitals in the U.S, suffering from COVID 19. The strain on the medical community was beyond belief, and became a crisis in almost every state, as no-where were facilities, and equipment prepared for the requirements and demands of the pandemic. Since November over 40% of the U.S. Hospitals have reached the breaking point. The ICU staffs are stressed, as they do their normal duties, change IV bags, monitor breathing apparatus, and are being pushed beyond human capabilities, with shorthanded staff. In the Southwest, where the rates continue to skyrocket, over 80,000 are hospitalized, many in intensive care crowded facilities, or makeshift accommodations. Staffing has become a logistic nightmare, with states bringing in nursing staff from outstate states, in a virtual bidding war for help. Reports of nurses with ICU credentials are being paid up to $6,000 per week in many areas. The Houston Methodist Hospital was offering an $8,000 bonus for staff retention.

As January 2021 nears its end, the world faced a race of mass immunizations of its population, and dealing with the spread of the new variants, while awaiting new, and adequate vaccine supplies. One health expert from the International WHO stated, we face a pandemic paradox. Vaccines on one hand offer remarkable hope, while on the other hand, the new variants are presenting greater uncertainty and risk.

As vaccines appear to offer a way out of the pandemic, concerns over supply shortages, threatened to deepen the crisis in many parts of the world. Competition to secure additional production, raised tensions among neighboring nations. The U.S which currently has over 25% of the world infected population, is under a new administration, and has made the COVID pandemic the number one national priority. Nationwide, vaccination plans are underway with committed communication to the states so that effective scheduling can be established. This is in complete contrast to the lack of planning from the former administration.

The race to inoculate citizens on both sides of the Atlantic, comes as scientists are moving to combat the new, and more contagious variants. The most recent one, first discovered in South Africa, appears to be resilient to some antibody treatments, and could thwart the current vaccines. The current vaccine suppliers, Pfizer and Moderna and Novavax indicate their vaccine still neutralizes the virus, but are aggressively attempting to develop a booster shot tailored to the new variant. While these companies attempt to meet the needs of the world, another company, Johnson and Johnson is rapidly seeking approvals on its vaccine product, which only needs one dosage. The current product has proven effective in the U.S with a 72% efficiency rate, but has not been as effective in South Africa, where results are currently a disappointing rate of 57% against the new variant, and it is aggressively expanding. A similar result has occurred in Britain, where the Novavax trials reached a 90% success rate in trial, while less than 50% in South African trials.

The Johnson and Johnson vaccine has an additional benefit, in addition to one dosage, it can survive with refrigeration for up to three weeks, making it a more manageable choice in remote parts of the world where the exotic variants apparently have a greater chance to develop. The U.S is hopeful the J&J entry proves effective and is quickly available, as it was part of the U.S warp speed program, and the U.S has a supply commitment for 100 million doses by July 2021. The 100 million doses are significant, as only one dose is required which doubles the rate of vaccinations available. J&J also has a new manufacturing facility in Baltimore to mass produce the vaccine.

The variants of the original Chinese COVID – 19 viruses discovered in Britain, and now South Africa, has infected people in seven Africa nations, as well as other countries confirming almost daily. It was most recently confirmed in the U.S, with two South Carolina residents infected with the new variant. The new more aggressive variants, coupled with increased travel, and COVID fatigue, have created a perfect storm for the new wave of infections. Countries have begun to react to this new spread, by banning travel and reinforcing restrictions. Germany for example, has banned travel from Brazil, Britain, Portugal and South Africa, beginning January 29th. In Hong Kong all returning air and sea crew members, are required to self-isolate in a quarantine hotel for 14 days, after which they will undergo seven days of medical surveillance

In China, a team of 10 scientists emerged from 10 days of quarantine in Wuhan, to begin work to establish the origins of the virus, which first appeared there in late 2019. This long-awaited investigation comes after months of politically charged negotiations between the Chinese Government and the WHO. It is set to include extensive interviews with the local scientists, health care workers, and workers at the seafood market deemed to be the origination point of the original outbreak. The U.S has taken a different role with the WHO, with the new administration, and looks forward to supporting its progress and documentation of the origin of the virus.

In a recent report released on Thursday January 28th 2021, from the Lowry Institute in Sydney, Australia where 100 countries were ranked on six measures of performance following each nation's handling of the pandemic for a thirty-six-week period, after that individual country reached its 100th confirmed case of COVID – 19

Out of 100 countries ranked, the US came in 94th.

February 2021

A year ago, when the outbreaks were in the beginning stages around the world, and uniform testing and reporting were inconsistent, the starting point for calculating what has transpired in one year is difficult to confirm. It took until July 2020 to reach 20 million infected cases, then 2 months later, it reached 40 million infected cases. It doubled by the end of 2020, then took one month to go from 80 to 100 million, by the end of January 2021. Beginning February 2021, the world had over 100 million case infections reported, with over 460,000 new cases reported in a one day, and over 13,800 deaths. The virus continues to sweep across the world, and very few places if any, have been able to avoid it.

Beginning in February 2021, the world was involved in massive vaccination procedures, while aggressively pursuing acquisition of available vaccines. Basically, worldwide there are three available for distribution, the Pfizer/BioNTech, Moderna, and Oxford/AstraZeneca. The Pfizer, and Moderna vaccines have been approved for use in the UK, Europe, and the U.S. The AstraZeneca has been approved in the UK and Europe, but awaits approval in the U.S. Each of these three vaccines require two dosages, and massive vaccination programs are underway worldwide. Russia has developed a vaccine, Sputnik 2, which is the current focus for their vaccination program. Likewise, China has developed vaccines, Sinovac, CanSino, and Sinopharm, which originated in China and they have made contract arrangements with other Asian countries, as well as South America.

The AstraZeneca vaccine reportedly, has not shown to maintain the same effectiveness level on the variant discovered in Africa, and the scientists at AstraZeneca are working to modify the current vaccine. The WHO suggests that as new variants surface, current vaccine effectiveness could be affected. The current vaccine from AstraZeneca, is seeking approval in the U.S.

The impact of new variants being discovered, has raised immense concern not only in the U.S, but worldwide. Initially it was the variant discovered in England that raised concern, but now we have other strains, that are impacting infection rates and virus control. In the U.S, studies have confirmed the UK variant is spreading rapidly, and significant community spreading may be occurring. Although it remains at low frequency, it is doubling every week and if similar to the progress in other countries, it would appear to be 35% to 45% more transmissible than earlier strains.

Johnson and Johnson have their Vaccine in Phase 3 clinical trials and will seek emergency approval targeted for the beginning of March 2021, and has production schedules to produce 100 million dosages in April of 2021. The Johnson and Johnson entry is currently the one which has advantageous refrigeration requirements, and requires only one dosage. Janssens and Novavax vaccines are also in Phase 3 trials

Worldwide, 171 Vaccines are currently in pre-clinical trials worldwide.

FEBRUARY 2021 CHALLENGES

As the world proceeds with COVID-19 and the path it continues to leave, some of the efforts appear to be one step forward, two steps back. In general, most countries face similar complicated issues, as the world attempts to control the virus.

1. The impact escalating daily of the new variants, with almost a guarantee, others are just around the corner. The variant discovered in Britain late 2020 (B 117) was discovered in the U.S in December, but further review suggests it probably arrived in November, and is spreading at an uncontrollable rate, doubling every 10 days. This could potentially bring a new surge, of hospitalizations and deaths. The CDC has warned the variant could become the dominant virus by March, if it follows a similar path as it did in England, Ireland, Portugal, and Jordon. The surges and control are much more complicated in the U.S, as the individual states have continued to manage the virus progress independently, as the previous administration had no Federal direction, and it raged out of control. The contagiousness of the B117, makes it a very serious threat. There is an uncertainty on the long-term effect of vaccines, and the impact of new variants could potentially create new hospitalization surges. The new virus entries also create uncertainties on individuals, who previous were infected and also vaccinated. Are they immune from reinfection of the new variants?

2. The variant from South Africa appears not to be responding to vaccinations from Astra Zeneca at the same level as the Pfizer and Moderna. As a result, officials announced suspension of vaccinations using the AstraZeneca's vaccine. AstraZeneca reportedly is working on updated versions, as are the other vaccine manufacturers. The producers face very difficult challenges, as new variants are bound to surface, and have possible different reactions to each virus.

3. Return to classroom instruction, is a decision every state in the U.S, and every country faces with great difficulty. Most states in the U.S had in classroom, or distance learning, or a combination of the two. Many school districts left decisions to the parents, when schools became open, or changed the regulations. As vaccinations became, and are becoming more available, school teachers are in the priority groups in most states, and many teachers are reluctant, or refuse to return unless they receive a vaccination. In addition, many teachers protest a return, until a safer environment exists, and their Unions are backing their efforts.

4. Countries continue to lock down, and return slowly to any normal process. Travel continues to be banned throughout Europe and virtually every country has strict procedures of control. In the U.S, a negative test is required from international travelers prior to entering the U.S.

The devastation created by the pandemic has impacted Companies and families throughout the world. In one years' time here in the U.S, over 450,000 people have died, leaving families in shock, and in many cases, financial ruin. The list of businesses that have not survived, continues to grow beyond belief. Worst yet, it's not over and won't be until vaccinations reach 75 – 80% of the population. The world remains at risk.

Life as we knew it, celebration of holidays, and family events, will never be the same. Worldwide families cling to memories, and pray this too shall pass.

Currently in the U.S. California has surpassed 43,000 COVID deaths to become the second state with a death count exceeding 43,000. 558 deaths were reported in one day, and 623 in the next, to put California on track to exceed the death count currently in New York. Vaccinations in California exceed all U.S. states with 1 million people being vaccinated in one week. Plans at the new Levi football stadium, will join other NFL stadiums to create vaccine sites, and the Levi stadium plans to vaccinate over 15,000 people per day.

While many areas continue with large infection rates, nationally the number of cases, hospitalization, and deaths, are beginning to decline nationwide. We have a four-week downward trend resulting in a 50% decline since the peak on January 8th. The U.S reported less than 100,000 cases for the first time since November 2nd of 2020. The hospital occupancy level also continues to decline to just over 81,000 hospitalized with COVID, the lowest patient count since November 19th 2020. 41 states are reporting a decline in the seven-day average of new COVID-19 cases while 9 are remaining essentially the same. This confirms the beginning of success of the vaccination effort as over 39,000,000 doses have been administered by February 10th with 9% of the population receiving one or more doses.

While the infection rate shows signs of slowing, the spread of the Variant from England is spreading rapidly throughout the U.S, doubling every 10 days. It is not known whether This UK. variant is more virulent or deadly, but it is more transmissible. The CDC warns that it could become the predominant virus in the U.S., if it spreads the way it did in the UK. Scientists are concerned about the effectiveness of this variant as well as its effectiveness against the South African variant and the impact of vaccination rates of success.

The worldwide vaccination impact is beginning to slow the massive spread of the pandemic. As production continues to increase on approved vaccines, and the possible addition of new vaccines, we are starting to see a light at the end of the tunnel. Many factors impact the progress throughout the world, such as reluctance by many to get a vaccination. There is a refusal for political, or religious beliefs, lack of facilities and or trained personnel, to manage in many of the 3rd world countries. Reviewing the % of the population that have been vaccinated around the world, there is a dramatic difference in the rate of progress by country.

If you review the vaccination doses administered per 100 people mid-February 2021, Israel by far leads the world in administering vaccinations to the residents of their country.

Cumulative COVID-19 vaccination doses per 100 people February 2021

COUNTRY	DOSES PER 100 PEOPLE
ISRAEL	79.48
UNITED ARAB REPUBLIC	53.43
UNITED KINGDOM	24.30
UNITED STATES	17.00
CHILE	12.43
EUROPEAN UNION	5.19
CHINA	2.82
BRAZIL	2.77
RUSSIA	2,67
MEXICO	0.96

It's obvious the ability to effectively manage the process, has major implications throughout the world. Also, again the data available from some of the countries lacks creditability, and reporting systems can have variance. But the progress of the vaccination effort has impacted the infection rate, and the death rate, the past 30 days 2021.

7 day rolling average January 17th   **7 day rolling average February 17th**

CASES	DEATH RATE	CASES DEATH RATE	CASES	CASES DEATH RATE
US	3,318	657	2,062	244
United Kingdom	1,123	682	584	182

Germany	852	205	437	87
France	362	280	382	282
India	180	11	93	8
Canada	147	183	62	80

By the middle of February 2021 at least seven different vaccines, have been rolled out to attack the original virus, and the new variants surfacing around the world. In December 2020, there were over 200 vaccine candidates for COVID-19 in development, with at least 52 in human trials.

As February 2021 comes to an end, and one year of record-breaking daily infections, death tolls are finally beginning to subside. Countries and scientists are seeing a light at the end of the tunnel. Beginning January, which on the 7th reached a record high of 844,324 new cases in one day, then began a steady reduction to 433,000 on February 26th. Vaccinations continue at a record pace in virtually every state and every country. Corresponding death rates and hospitalizations confirm the effectiveness of the vaccine effort. While Pfizer and Moderna continue to be the two major vaccines, Astra Zeneca has been approved in many countries, as well as vaccine entries from Russia and China. The U.S has by the end of February received FDA approval of the Johnson and Johnson vaccine. This new vaccine does not currently record the success rate of the two previous approved vaccines, but for worldwide distribution, it has major advantages with requiring only one shot, and a huge refrigeration benefit, not requiring freezing levels to maintain. The benefit of these issues makes this much easier in a vaccination effort for third world countries. In addition, the addition of another major vaccine added to the supply train gives the vaccination rate a huge boost and brings the control efforts closer to reality.

March 2021

The Johnson and Johnson vaccine arrived the first week in March and provides a much-anticipated addition to the vaccination pro-cess worldwide. In the U.S., new vaccination facilities were opening as the supply of vaccines were now becoming more readily available and in increased quantities. The Johnson and Johnson approved vaccine presents an advantage to many areas by requiring only one dosage. Rural farming communities who would be required to drive a long distance, and be away from needs on the farm, see this as a benefit. The ability to be able accommodate homeless, with only one dosage, as well as people without a personal physician or medical connection. Smaller Pharmacies in rural communities who would not be able to meet the refrigeration requirements of the original two approved vaccines, and schools and plant facilities who would be faced with time off requirements of two shots versus one. Also, in the minority communities who tend to resist vaccinations, it becomes much easier to sell individuals on doing it once, rather than attempting to schedule a second vaccination.

The perception of the new Johnson and Johnson addition, in the U.S., versus the Pfizer and Moderna, does present a challenge when and if the Johnson and Johnson vaccine becomes visualized as an inferior choice due to its perceived emphasis in minority groups, and for the less fortunate. All attempts are being made to emphasize the benefits of receiving a vaccination rather than viewing the choices as a Luxury or non-Luxury offering. At this stage of the immunization process, no one or two vaccines, have any clinical advantage

The vaccination process is expanding worldwide with great control progress. Worldwide by mid-march 10 vaccines around the world are being administered to reduce the growing threat of infections. Since the high point of infections around January 11th 2021, with a seven-day moving average of 249,360 case infections being reported. There has been an overall decline of 79.4 % of the 7-day moving average since that 7-day high. Current 7 day moving average rates are 62,555 cs being reported March 2nd. The U.S vaccination program which began on December 14th 2020, is reporting 82.6 million vaccine doses have been administered. 16.3% of the U.S. population, have received at least one dose. These numbers will increase dramatically with the J&J addition. The dramatic impact of the vaccination process, is relieving the pressure on our health community which had been driven to the brink. Current hospitalization admissions decreased by 67 % from the 7 day rolling perks in mid-January. Daily admissions are falling by over 24%.

Deaths obviously are also declining as a result of the vaccine progress. There has been a 43% decline in the 7-day rolling daily death rate from the mid-January 7 day rolling averages. An example of the progress of the vaccination success in reducing deaths was in the U.S. where Minnesota reported the first day since early April 2020, where no Covid deaths were reported.

As signs of control appear to be well underway, the response by residents particularly in the U.S are of great concern to scientists and the health community. People in many cases, are resisting vaccinations, stating religious and or other concerns, and reduces the potential success of a massive coordinated effort to vaccinate a high % of the residents. People chose to ignore the controls which have gotten the world to this control level, and could easily begin a new increase in the expanse of the virus, especially with the massive expansion of new variants currently gaining ground, and possible additional variants which are unknown as we enter year 2 of Covid. Also of concern is the success of the vaccinations that have been given to elderly, and others, to contain the variants currently being spread, and possible new ones on the horizon. Scientists and health officials want things to begin to normalize but with caution and control to protect others.

As March progresses, schools are opening, restaurants are approving new capacity levels, and entertainment facilities are looking to open at managed attendance levels. Worldwide travel is being opened with caution. As the world begins to reduce restrictions beginning March, it comes with a very high risk. The past two weeks in March have seen increased infection and death rates, brought to a large extent by the new variants, which spread easily and presents a new challenge to the impact of current vaccinations long term success. When the world was viewing March 2020 as a new beginning, many issues surface as scientists attempt to understand the pandemic itself. New variants which began in England and South Africa, have spread dramatically throughout the world, and appear to spread more rapidly, and possibly are more deadly. As vaccines appear to have success in managing these new variants, its apparent we have not seen the last on new strains to control.

The world has faced a challenge, with universal implications. The need for worldwide cooperation and data transmission, has never been more evident than the need expressed this past year.

The failure of the U.S Administration in 2020, cost hundreds of thousands of lives, and impacted innocent families beyond imagination. The new administration appears to have taken this seriously, and is aggressively developing vaccination programs. Current effort is to Vaccinate 100 million in the 1st 100 days of the new administration. This new attitude is welcome news to most Americans, and the goal of 100 million was surpassed earlier than projected. The timetable requirements for individuals eligible for vaccination, continues to be moved forward with expectations now for all individuals desiring vaccinations completed by early summer. The problem continues to surface with Ex-President Trump's support group, who resist getting the vaccination and put people at risk shamelessly, without regard for others.

The worldwide vaccination campaign is the largest in history, By the middle of March 433 million doses have been administered in 133 countries. The latest rate is approximately 10.7 million per day. In the U.S. 124 million doses have been administered.

While 433 million doses are a staggering number, it represents only 2.8% of the global population. At the current rate of 10 to 11 million per day, it would take years to vaccinate the entire world. Countries like Israel and the UK have made tremendous strides in leading the world in vaccinations, but the world continues to be in a life and death race, between vaccines and virus. New vaccines will undoubtedly be produced and the likelihood of new variants will also raise new challenges.

April 2022

Beginning April much progress is being made, but in much of the world, its one step forward, and two steps backward. Spring break, flooding the beaches in worldwide vacation resorts after months of confinement with little regard to protect others. Masks and social distancing were totally disregarded, and many new infections will return as the college students return home. A new wave is expected with the expanded travel and freedom. Add to these threats, potential protesting, and a refusal to be vaccinated by the far-right people of the U.S. Many of these are intelligent people, who refuse to come to grips with any sense of responsibility, or concern for other people. Hopefully it doesn't take a death of a loved family member for those to get the message.

The 2nd year appears to give us a light at the end of the tunnel. The more people who get vaccinated the brighter the light at the end of the tunnel becomes. Those who have no concern for others, and lack common sense, will contribute to a dark uncontrolled progression of needless deaths. This coupled with expansion of the new variants, will dim the anticipated the light, the world continues to pray for.

The impact of COVID while making great strides will have its impact felt for years and possibly generations, Millions have lost their jobs, the downtown business structure has been hollowed out as employees are working remotely, emptying the offices and putting a closure on retailers. Many never to reopen.

School shutdowns have contributed to a widened achievement gap, as many low-income families lacked the necessary technology to compete with affluent families. The gap between the haves and the have nots will widen as a result of the effects of COVID.

With a struggling world beginning of the 2nd year of the pandemic, the world is better prepared to manage case infections, new variant additions, and new control systems of vaccines.

The world has never seen a crisis of this magnitude which spared no part of the world, or people of the world.

2020 was.

TORN BY COVID

POSTSCRIPT

Indicated earlier was that the Pandemic presented the worldwide community with a unique opportunity to work as one society to contain the Pandemic, and in the process, reflect worldwide concern for others. It gave the worldwide community an opportunity to assure the third world countries it would have equal access to vaccines, and medical assistance to facilitate vaccinations. The WHO had proposed a plan of sharing development. and making vaccines available equally at no cost to all parts of the world. Unfortunately, greed raises its ugly head, and the U.S, UK, Russia, and China, the world powers with the resources, had control of the Pharma companies and contracted for basically the bulk of production, and do not appear to share a worldwide concern to share information, or assist the development countries in conquering and controlling this pandemic. Third world countries have extremely low vaccination rates, poor health control systems, and are struggling to obtain the needed vaccines to meet the needs of their population. This, while the wealthy nations continue to control the supplies.

It would be the hope of the people of the world, that we can usually find some good, even when all appears bad. We share a common crisis. We share a common concern for other nations, even if was a selfish concern, that their misfortunes could benefit us, with their continued intelligence and communication. Hopefully we can find a way through this tragic event to share a common goal. We live as humans, hopefully with a purpose during our lifetimes. We have a chance to better understand each other, and work towards being a resource to our fellow man. Our faith needs to spill over to help other inhabitants living with us in our world community.

Torn by 2020, we see light for future generations at the end of the tunnel.

THE WRITER

2020 WAS A YEAR TORN BY PANDEMIC

The data outlined in this manuscript has evolved from numerous sources such as the daily paper, the CDC recaps, WHO tracking, and various computer on line sources. Any errors or miscalculations are misinterpretations by the writer.

Epilogue

As April 2021 progressed after the 2020 Torn Journal, tremendous progress was being made worldwide vaccinating the public which resulted in major declines in COVID infections Hospitalizations and deaths. The addition of the Johnson and Johnson vaccine gave a huge boost to the vaccine supply chain, and vaccinations began to open up for people of all ages over 16. While this new vaccine addition was being greeted with great enthusiasm, 6 people developed blood clouts and a hold was put on any further vaccinations of the Johnson and Johnson vaccine until studies could determine the cause, and the future for this vaccine. By April 24th, most countries had revised the suspensions, and the vaccine has been cleared for use with precautions.

While the vaccination process appeared to be making significant headway in beginning to control this disease, new surges in the rate of infections, in many countries along with the resulting numbers of deaths have the worldwide community with deep concern. As the Month of April draws to a close, the light at the end of the tunnel we thought was getting very close, presents many new concerns as reality sets in for mankind.

India is currently recording the highest daily infection totals of any country since the beginning of the pandemic, surpassing even the high totals previously recorded in the US. In one 24-hour period over 314,000 cases were recorded, bringing hospital availability to a standstill. Patients were forced to share beds and oxygen supplies were exhausted with no relief in sight. In one of the largest hospitals in Delhi, people were dying on the pavement outside of the hospital entrance, as there was nowhere to put them inside.

Clearly the pandemic is far from over, with 149.9 million people infected by late April 2021 and 3.1 million deaths being reported. Clearly the numbers are significantly higher, but the information from China is controlled, and not representative of actual data.

As vaccinations worldwide make significant progress, so too does the need for personal responsibility. In the U.S. People have become careless, events are beginning to reopen, too many of the residents are refusing shots, which impacts others and the seriousness of the pandemic is being ignored. This while the new variants are driving new infections at record levels. Unless the people of the world accept how critical this situation is, and respond as concerned humans, we will face another 2020, torn by pandemic.

CPSIA information can be obtained
at www.ICGtesting.com
Printed in the USA
BVHW052006190423
662664BV00002B/31